Treating Suicidal Behavior

TREATMENT MANUALS FOR PRACTITIONERS
David Barlow, *Editor*

Treating Suicidal Behavior

An Effective, Time-Limited Approach

M. DAVID RUDD
THOMAS JOINER
M. HASAN RAJAB

Series Editor's Note by David H. Barlow

THE GUILFORD PRESS
New York   London

*To my wife, Loretta, and two children—Nicholas and Emma—
who remind me on a daily basis of the simple but wonderful things
that make life so meaningful.*

—M. DAVID RUDD

To my mother and sisters, and in memory of my dad.

—THOMAS JOINER

© 2001 The Guilford Press
A Division of Guilford Publications, Inc.
72 Spring Street, New York, NY 10012
www.guilford.com

Printed in the United States of America

This book is printed on acid-free paper.

Last digit is print number: 9   8   7   6   5   4   3   2   1

Library of Congress Cataloging-in-Publication Data

Rudd, M. David
    Treating sucidial behavior: an effective, time-limited approach /
M. David Rudd, Thomas Joiner, M. Hasan Rajab.
        p. cm. — (Treatment manuals for practitioners)
    Includes bibliographical references and index.
    ISBN 1-57230-614-9 (hardcover)
        1. Sucidial behavior—Treatment.   2. Suicide—Prevention.   I. Joiner,
Thomas E.   II. Rajab, M. Hasan.   III. Title.   IV. Series.
RC569 .R83 2000
616.85′844506—dc21

                                                                00-045474

About the Authors

M. David Rudd, PhD, ABPP, is Professor of Psychology and Director of Clinical Training at Baylor University. He completed is doctoral training at the University of Texas at Austin and completed postdoctoral training at the Beck Institute in Philadelphia. In addition to training, he maintains a part-time private practice. He has authored over 60 articles and book chapters, many addressing the issue of suicidality. His work has been recognized by the American Association of Suicidology (1999 Recipient of the Edwin Shneidman Award) and the Texas Psychological Association (1998 Outstanding Contribution to Science Award). He also serves as the Chair of the Texas State Board of Examiners of Psychologists.

Thomas Joiner, PhD, is Professor of Pscyhology and Director of the Psychology Clinic at Florida State University. He completed his doctoral training at the University of Texas at Austin. Dr. Joiner has authored over 100 articles and book chapters in the areas of depression, eating disorders, and suicidality. Dr. Joiner's work has received broad acclaim for his impact on the field, including the David Shakow Early Career Award for Distinguished Scientific Contribution from the Division of Clinical Psychology of the American Psychological Association in 1997 and the APA Early Career Award for Psychopathology Research in 2000.

M. Hasan Rajab, PhD, is Associate Professor in the Department of Psychiatry and Behavioral Science at Texas A&M Health Science Center. Dr. Rajab completed his doctoral training in biostatistics at Texas A&M University. He is the author of several articles addressing a range of issues in methodology and biostatistics.

100221

Series Editor Note

No problem facing clinicians is more urgent than suicidal behavior. Data continue to indicate that suicide remains one of the leading causes of death in our younger population, and is on the increase. And yet, clinicians are surprisingly ill equipped to deal with this most profound of all human problems. While organized and manualized treatment approaches exist for syndromes with which suicide is strongly associated, such as depression and borderline personality disorder, no empirically based strategies have been available targeting suicidal behavior directly and specifically. Now, M. David Rudd, Thomas Joiner, and M. Hasan Rajab provide such a tool. In so doing, they offer clinicians for the first time a flexible and unique therapeutic program that is direct, time-limited, and buttressed by empirical support. Thus, clinicians facing the urgency of suicidal behavior can decide on the content and timing of interventions designed to eliminate suicidal behavior, and assess in an ongoing way the effectiveness of their efforts. Even if not often confronted with suicidal behavior, clinicians who become familiar with the procedures outlined in this manual will gain confidence in their ability to deal with suicidal crises.

DAVID H. BARLOW

Preface

Treating Suicidality: A Brief Overview

Over the last decade, the assessment and treatment of suicidal behavior has received increasing attention in day-to-day clinical practice. This trend is likely the result of a number of identifiable factors:

1. The exponential increase in malpractice claims brought against care providers in cases of both inpatient and outpatient suicide (e.g., Jobes & Berman, 1993).
2. The emergence of ethical guidelines defining and mandating specific training, clinical experience, and areas of competence in working with suicidal patients (e.g., Bongar, 1992; Bongar & Harmatz, 1989; Kleespies, 1993).
3. Refinement in applied and research nomenclature in suicidology (O'Carroll et al., 1996).
4. The recent publication of initial inpatient and outpatient standards of care (Bongar, Maris, Berman, & Litman, 1992; Bongar, Maris, Berman, Litman, & Silverman, 1993; Silverman, Berman, Bongar, Litman, & Maris, 1994).

The net result of this convergence of factors has essentially been threefold. First, there is a heightened level of awareness of the complexity of the issues clinicians face when working with suicidal patients, clinically, ethically, and legally. Second, there is increasing recognition of the specific, identifiable tasks of assessment and treatment that are unique to working with suicidal patients and invariable regardless of the psychotherapeutic orientation employed. And third, clinicians have become more acutely aware of the limitations in existing research in suicidality. There is limited empirical support for much of what is routine in the clinical practice of assessment and treatment; this absence highlights the need for a clear, rational, and organized approach.

The increased attention garnered by suicidality over the last decade has been coupled with dramatic changes in the nature of the health care delivery system. Managed care has dramatically changed the way in which we practice psychotherapy (i.e., what we actually do, how often we do it, and the time frame for which we can continue). This is the case even with the most difficult patients. Suicide shows no signs of being eliminated or reduced as a public health threat, particularly for 10- to 44-year-olds. Suicide ranks as one of the leading causes of death for those 10 years of age and older and the number of attempts is estimated to range anywhere from 8 to 25 for every completion (National Institute of Mental Health, 1998). For some, long-term therapy is a thing of the past, at least in the traditional sense of the word (e.g., Nathan, 1998; Seligman, 1996).

In all likelihood, most of us will be treating suicidal patients on a more regular basis, with fewer resources, and under more severe time constraints, despite severely limited efficacy data and the lack of any consensus about what actually works in treatment (see Chapter 1, this volume). This book is intended to provide a manual for time-limited treatment, one that is empirically based while simultaneously recognizing and acknowledging the constraints and limitations faced in psychotherapy practice in the 21st century.

Never before have issues of time, money, and documented outcome been so prominent in discussions about appropriate risk assessment, management, and treatment. All too often, clinicians today find themselves asking, "How can I treat this patient safely and effectively in the time we've been given?" Clinicians also find themselves asking questions such as, "How will I know things are working?" In response, many have turned to treatment manuals in an effort to adapt to the unique pressures of working under severe time limitations with complex clinical problems (Lambert, 1998). Whether or not this is actually a good outcome has been hotly debated, with contentious arguments on both sides.

Implications of a Treatment Manual for Suicidality

The use of manuals in the treatment of suicidality has not been commonplace. Actually, other than Linehan's (1993) dialectical behavior therapy targeting borderline personality disorder, no other manuals exist that specifically target suicidality. Although some of the arguments made about treatment manuals in general can be applied to this one, it is believed that the advantages far out-weigh the disadvantages (e.g., Craighead & Craighead, 1998; Kendall, 1998; Lambert, 1998). We believe that we offer the clinician something quite unique: an empirically based manual with a strong theoretical framework that is realistically flexible, one that relies on the clinician's judgment, skill, and expertise for effective implementation. We hope to offer the clinician a treatment manual that helps answer some of the fundamental questions we face every day in our offices, ones complicated by the diagnostic and interpersonal complexity presented by suicidal patients:

- What is the nature of the problem (i.e., diagnosis and risk assessment)?
- What needs to be done (i.e., clinical intervention)?
- When is it best to do it (i.e., treatment sequence and timing)?
- How do I know if it is working (i.e., assessing treatment outcome)?

The treatment approach presented here is, without doubt, a structured, manualized approach. But we also believe that it is unique for a number of reasons. First, we provide a solid, theoretically based treatment with empiri-cal support that can be applied in time-limited settings. Second, as will be-come apparent in reading this book, the approach is still flexible enough for day-to-day clinical practice with complex and challenging comorbid disor-ders that are commonplace in suicidality. Accordingly, the treatment model is ideal for treatment effectiveness studies, which have been called for in an effort to complement and balance initial controlled clinical trials and related efficacy studies (e.g., Seligman, 1996). Third, the treatment model offered not only recognizes but also emphasizes the critical importance of the thera-peutic relationship and therapist-specific variables in treating suicidality. Fourth, it also recognizes the importance of interpersonal process in be-havioral change with this population. And fifth, the treatment framework offered depends on careful monitoring of risk and related treatment out-come, consistent with the elaboration of others on the importance of system-atic monitoring of treatment outcome for all psychotherapy patients (e.g., Lambert & Okiishi, 1997).

All in all, we believe we have put together a treatment manual that cuts across all aspects of treating suicidal behavior. It is one well suited for today's unique treatment environment. It is a framework that can be applied over the long term, but one uniquely designed for time-limited care. It is one that is structured but paradoxically flexible. In the end, though, it is a manual that provides the clinician with a comprehensive framework for the assessment, management, and psychotherapeutic treatment of the suicidal patient.

Structure of the Treatment Manual

We have organized the book in two sections. The first lays out the theoretical and empirical foundation. The second covers the specific tasks involved in assessment and treatment. We have tried to be comprehensive and to incorporate case conceptualization, risk assessment, crisis intervention, treatment planning and specific treatment targets, and the monitoring of treatment outcome. We also address a range of special topics and considerations such as the role of group treatment, the use of medications, patient selection, and termination of treatment. We hope readers will find more than ample information on how to effectively treat suicidal behavior within a time-limited world but likewise find the approach amenable to individual nuances, clinical creativity, and varying levels of skill, training, and experience.

Acknowledgments

David Rudd wishes to thank Jay Burke for providing a supportive work environment rich with opportunity for intellectual growth; Dave Stulman, Betty Clark, and Gary Brooks for their support and friendship; Harry Rumzek and Tammy Delvecchio for providing able and eager assistance even with some of the more mundane and tedious tasks; Thomas Joiner for his scientific rigor and simple brilliance and for being a friend and collaborator; and, most important, Loretta, Nicholas, and Emma, who have given my life unwavering perspective and value.

Thomas Joiner wishes to thank the faculty, graduate students, and staff of the Department of Psychology at Florida State University for a scholarly, stimulating, and collegial atmosphere; David Rudd for initiation into suicidology and for collaboration and friendship; and, especially, Malachi and Graciela for love and patience, and for putting even something as important as treating suicide in its proper place.

M. DAVID RUDD
THOMAS JOINER
M. HASAN RAJAB

Contents

3. An Overview of the Treatment Process   44

II. ASSESSMENT AND TREATMENT

4. Treatment Course and Session-by-Session Guidelines   79

5. The Evaluation Process and the Initial Interviews   100

I

ESTABLISHING A FOUNDATION FOR TREATMENT

1

What Do We Really Know
about Treating Suicidality?:
A Critical Review of the Literature

What do we really know about treating suicidality? In other words, what works, under what conditions, and for whom? To answer these questions with some degree of accuracy we need to rely on scientific data, regardless of the depth or breadth of the literature. Otherwise, we are left to conclusions based on speculation and supposition, two demons that have plagued those practicing psychotherapy in today's managed care environment. More than ever before, clinicians are being asked to do more with less and to treat complex disorders in time-limited fashion. Under such conditions, an empirical foundation to practice is essential for safe, effective, and appropriate treatment, particularly for those presenting with suicidality. In short, we need to have *reasonable* expectations for recovery. Identifying reasonable expectations, essential treatment targets, and minimal duration of care is, for the most part, an empirical challenge that can only be answered through the application of science.

There are some suicidal individuals who simply will not be effectively treated over the short term, those who present with chronic and severe psychopathology. It is crucial that we make a coherent argument grounded in science when asked the question, Why not? Others will make considerable progress, never making another suicide attempt, and if subsequent suicidal cri-

Portions of this chapter previously appeared in Rudd (2000). Copyright 2000 by The Guilford Press. Adapted by permission.

ses arise, they will be effectively diffused. Again, it is crucial that we make a coherent argument grounded in science when asked the question, Why?

In reviewing the literature that addresses the psychotherapeutic treatment of suicidality, a number of important questions surface. Among them are the following:

- What treatments have been demonstrated effective for suicidality?
- Within identified treatments, are there common *core interventions* associated with positive outcome?
- Are there identified treatments that clearly should *not* be used as a result of consistently poor outcome data?
- Can high-risk suicidal patients be treated safely *and* effectively on an outpatient basis?
- Are there prohibitive features of particular treatments such as exorbitant costs, duration, frequency, intensity, risks, or side effects?
- Are there differential dropout rates for specific treatment approaches that need to be considered?
- Does treatment setting influence outcome (i.e., inpatient, outpatient, partial hospitalization, residential, and day treatment)?
- Does treatment *delay* (i.e., the period of time from suicidal crisis to the onset of treatment) predict treatment outcome?
- Is treatment duration associated with outcome? That is, are short-term treatments more or less effective than longer ones?
- Do particular subgroups (e.g., multiple attempters) require specific treatment approaches with unique variations?
- Does treatment effect endure? That is, what are the observed relapse rates?
- Are there identified approaches specifically targeting those that relapse? Likewise, are relapse prevention programs effective?
- Does diagnostic comorbidity affect treatment selection, prognosis, or outcome (i.e., treatment matching)?

As will become evident in the following review, we can answer only a few of the most fundamental questions raised regarding the treatment of suicidality. And at that, our answers are tentative. They do, nonetheless, provide an empirically derived set of conclusions on which to build. Additional answers depend on continued growth in the science of clinical suicidology, collegial debate and discussion, and the creative evolution of psychotherapy.

The Available Literature: A Limited Database

Although a large number of studies exist in the suicidality literature, incorporating case examples, theoretical articles, and studies without comparison or control groups, our review includes only those that are randomized or controlled in some fashion. This is consistent with our original goal of integrating existing science into practice in suicidality, as well as articulating and acknowledging current limitations in the state of the science. By doing so, we can articulate an empirically grounded approach to practice, appropriately acknowledge significant and surprising limitations in this area of scientific study, and identify questions that need to be answered.

A thorough review of the literature (*PsycINFO* and *MEDLINE*) yielded a total of 25 randomized or controlled studies targeting suicidality (see Rudd, 2000, for a detailed summary of all studies). None are specific to adolescents, although a few include older adolescents (i.e., ages 17–19) and young adults. This total incorporates both intervention and treatment studies. Those classified as intervention studies (i.e., $n = 6$) included those that were specifically described as not providing any identifiable form of psychotherapy as the study condition. These studies essentially made procedural changes in both the provision of and ease of access to traditional psychotherapeutic services, exploring any subsequent reduction in suicide attempts. All were careful to note that the study condition was not psychotherapeutic treatment, although several faced considerable confounds. Among the studies reviewed, interventions varied but included the following: (1) supportive case management by volunteer workers (Termansen & Bywater, 1975), (2) simple follow-up letters and phone calls to those refusing treatment (Motto, 1976), (3) incorporation of home visits and more intensive tracking (Litman & Wold, 1976; Van Heeringen et al., 1995), (4) brief medical hospitalization with no psychiatric care whatsoever (Waterhouse & Platt, 1990), and (5) improved ease of access to 24-hour emergency services (Morgan, Jones, & Owen, 1993).

Of the 25 studies identified, three explored pharmacological treatment of suicidality and were excluded from our review given that the focus is on psychotherapeutic treatment (Hirsch, Walsh, & Draper, 1983; Montgomery & Montgomery, 1982; Montgomery, Roy, & Montgomery, 1981). It is interesting to note that the three pharmacological studies were all completed over two decades ago, prior to some of the recent advances in the use of medications for diagnosed psychiatric disorders, particularly selective serotonin reuptake inhibitors (SSRIs). This highlights a common problem in the scientific study of suicidality; those evidencing some form of suicidality are ordinarily excluded from clinical trials, both medication and psychotherapy, due to their high-risk nature. After excluding the three medication studies, we were left with a total of 22 controlled or randomized studies targeting the treatment of suicidality. This is consistent with a recent review of outcome studies offered by Linehan (1997). Our total includes three studies not previously reviewed (i.e., Joiner, Rudd, & Rajab, 1998b; Lerner & Clum, 1990; Rudd, Rajab, et al., 1996b). As noted previously, this total includes six simple *intervention* studies, not purporting to address more complex psychotherapeutic treatment issues, which leaves only 16 treatment studies for critical review, a truly surprising finding for any area of science, not to mention one fraught with so much controversy and importance.

A Critical Review of Intervention Studies: Do Simple Procedural Changes Make a Difference?

Of the intervention studies reviewed, three had positive findings, but each has identifiable limitations, some which are considerable. Termansen and Bywater (1975) found that what essentially was described as *intensive case management* by volunteer workers reduced subsequent suicide attempts during the 3-month follow-up period, relative to those receiving no follow-up care. As the authors noted, "the role [of the volunteers] was not therapeutic in the conventional psychiatric sense; rather it was the role of the helper expressing concern for the person in his total environmental situation" (p. 29). The study included four conditions, with each varying as to the nature of initial assessment and follow-up monitoring. The first group was assessed in the emergency room after a suicide attempt. They also received follow-up intervention by a mental health worker for a total of 3 months. The second group was also assessed in the emergency room after an attempt but did not receive intensive intervention. They were, however, provided follow-up at a crisis center as needed. The third and fourth groups received no follow-up care of any type and served as controls, with the third receiving initial intervention in the emergency room and the fourth no initial intervention.

The findings are compromised by the fact that the intervention was poorly defined in both content and application. What actually was done is highly questionable. Whether the intervention was *psychotherapy* is also arguable. Further, the experimental and comparison groups were not comparable at intake, a confound that renders interpretation of results questionable if not impossible. Also, the follow-up period was inordinately brief, rendering the results of limited practical value. Finally, standardized outcome measures were not used, there was a relatively high attrition rate (37%), suicide intent was not assessed at intake and prior to randomization, and no exclusion criteria were stated. In light of the brief follow-up period noted and the considerable methodological problems cited, the findings reported by Termansen and Bywater (1975) have questionable utility and practical application.

Similar to the goal of Termansen and Bywater (1975), Van Heerignen et al. (1995) explored the use of home visits by a community nurse in enhancing treatment compliance and reducing subsequent attempts in comparison to *usual outpatient care* (i.e., without home visits targeting treatment compliance). The intervention was fairly simple in nature and described as follows: "during the home visits reasons for non-compliance were assessed, needs for treatment evaluated and identified needs matched with the supply of outpatient treatment" (p. 964). Findings revealed better treatment compliance among those in the experimental group and, although not significant, a favorable trend (p = .056) was noted in the reduction of subsequent attempts at 1 year. Although the attrition rate was 24%, the study was relatively well designed for its stated purpose, posing no severe methodological problems that would undermine the fundamental conclusions noted. The study did, however, exclude the highest-risk cases, limiting the utility of the findings. In addition, the *mechanism of action* for the home visits was not interpretable. The actual nature of the intervention during the home visits was not directed by a standard protocol, nor were intervention process variables and related data collected. As a result, we are left to conclude that home visits improved compliance but can only speculate as to how or why.

In another relatively well-designed study for its stated purpose, Morgan et al. (1993) found that improved ease of access to 24-hour emergency services over the period of a year following a first suicide attempt significantly reduced subsequent attempts among those in the experimental group relative to those receiving management as usual after an attempt (i.e., ranging from inpatient psychiatric admission to referral back to the primary care physician). In somewhat elegant fashion, improved ease of access was accomplished simply by giving the patient a "green card" with emergency numbers and encouragement to seek services early in a crisis by going to the emergency room, calling by telephone, or seeking emergency admission. The authors hoped to target the specific problem of low treatment compliance among first-time attempters. Interestingly and paradoxically, they also found that this simple procedural change also significantly reduced service demand in the experimental group. Perhaps the primary limitation of the study was the fact that it targeted first-time attempters, excluding the highest-risk group, that is, those making multiple attempts and experiencing chronic suicidality.

Among negative intervention findings, Motto (1976) found that simple follow-up letters and telephone calls to those refusing treatment after presenting in crisis did not reduce suicide rates over a 4-year follow-up period, although a favorable trend was observed. This finding is not particularly surprising. Actually, what is surprising is that investigators noted an encouraging trend after 4 years, with fewer suicides among those receiving the simple follow-up contacts. Litman and Wold (1976) found that telephone calls, home visits, and *befriending contacts* (i.e., what was termed "continuing relationship maintenance") by crisis volunteers did not reduce the frequency of suicide attempts in the experimental group over a period of 24 months, despite an improvement in quality of life. Litman and Wold (1976) were careful to note that "the service was not considered therapy" (p. 531). Although negative, the findings reported by Litman and Wold (1976) are compromised by considerable methodological problems and, as a result, are questionable if not simply uninterpretable. Among the problems are (1) a poorly defined intervention in type, duration, content, frequency, and monitoring; (2) acknowledgment of considerable overlap between the experimental and control conditions approaching equivalence and nullifying the results; (3) integration of individual and group meetings in the intervention group raising questions about the actual provision of therapy; (4) failure to define and implement uniform inclusion criteria for high-risk; (5) no stated exclusion criteria; and (6) lack of standardized outcome measures.

As previously, the negative findings reported by Waterhouse and Platt (1990) are also questionable. The stated purpose of the study was to evaluate the usefulness of simple and brief medical hospitalization (i.e., with no psychiatric care of any type provided) by nonpsychiatric staff at reducing subsequent attempts over the next 4 months. The control group was simply discharged to home. The average duration of the hospitalization for those in the experimental group was less than a day (i.e., 17 hours), and, accordingly, it is not surprising that no subsequent differences were observed in attempts between groups. The two groups were essentially comparable. In addition, the study targeted only those identified as low risk (i.e., further suicidal risk was assessed as low), raising questions as to the actual utility of the finding for clinical practice.

Implications for Clinical Practice

As is evident from the previous discussion, the intervention studies available allow for only a few tentative conclusions regarding interventions involved in the psychotherapeutic treatment and clinical management of suicidal patients. There is a considerable gap in the literature when it comes to a discussion of the interventions helpful with those at highest risk (i.e., chronic multiple attempters). At this point, we simply do not know what interventions are effective for this group. Following are some conclusions with limited empirical support:

1. Intensive follow-up, case management, telephone contacts, letters, or home visits may improve treatment compliance over the short term for lower-risk cases.
2. Improved ease of access (i.e., a clearly stated crisis plan) to emergency services can potentially reduce subsequent attempts and service demand by first-time suicide attempters.

A Critical Review of Treatment Studies:
An Emerging Trend for Cognitive-Behavioral Therapy

The treatment studies ($n = 16$) available that address suicidality can be divided into two broad categories: those providing short-term treatment (i.e., less than 6 months, $n = 14$) and those providing longer-term therapy (i.e., 6 months or greater, $n = 2$). Of the total, the results have been decidedly mixed, with eight rendering positive results about the efficacy of the treatment and six negative. However, among those with positive findings, the results are fairly consistent. Among the short-term studies, the majority ($n = 10$) offered some variant of a cognitive-behavioral therapy (CBT), each integrating a problem-solving component in some form or fashion as a *core intervention*. This is not particularly surprising given that CBT is perhaps the approach most amenable to a brief format. The duration of treatment varied across the CBT studies but ranged from a low of only 10 days (Liberman & Eckman, 1981) to a high of 3 months (Gibbons, Butler, Urwin, & Gibbons, 1978). It is important to note that two of the studies actually used the same sample (Joiner et al., 1998b; Rudd, Rajab, et al., 1996), resulting in a total of nine unique study samples on which to base conclusions about the efficacy of time-limited CBT (i.e., with a problem-solving *core* component) for suicidality.

Of the remaining four studies that fall within the brief treatment category, three explored the utility of what can be best described as an *additive component* to treatment as usual, that is, intensive follow-up care of some type, rather than the specific treatment modality (Chowdhury, Hicks, & Kreitman, 1973; Hawton et al., 1981; Welu, 1977). These studies cannot be classified as intervention studies, however, given the impossibility of differentiating the intervention from the actual treatment as the two were inextricably intertwined. One explored the impact of improved *continuity of care* on subsequent suicide attempts (Moeller, 1989). The study by van der Sande, Rooijen, Buskens, Allart, Hawton, van der Graaf, and Van Engeland (1997) had *additive features* (i.e., improved access to emergency services and home visits when necessary), but the stated purpose was to test *a crisis intervention approach for suicide attempters*, one that integrated problem solving training as the psychotherapeutic tool. Accordingly, it has been classified with the short-term treatment studies.

Of those studies addressing what was essentially an additive component to short-term treatment (i.e., more intensive follow-up), results were fairly negative. Both studies targeting intensive short term follow-up using a combination of home visits, telephone contact, and more frequent and flexible routine treatment appointments found no appreciable impact on subsequent suicide attempts over periods ranging from 6 to 12 months (Gibbons et al., 1978; Hawton et al., 1981). Hawton et al. (1981), not surprisingly, found that home visits did improve treatment compliance, in contrast to those receiving weekly outpatient care. Improved compliance did not, however, translate to a significant reduction in subsequent attempts over the 12-month follow-up period (i.e., 10% with subsequent attempts for those receiving home visits vs. 15% for traditional outpatients). Similarly, Chowdhury et al. (1973) found that home visits, more frequent outpatient appointments, and improved access to emergency services did not reduce subsequent attempts among multiple attempters in contrast to *treatment as usual*. Those receiving the experimental intervention did, however, report an improved *psychiatric and social status*. Not surprisingly, Moeller (1989) found that efforts to improve the *continuity of care* by assigning the same clinician before and after hospitalization had no appreciable impact on suicide attempts during the yearlong follow-up period.

In contrast, Welu (1977), in a well-designed study, found that more intensive follow-up using home visits, telephone contact, and more frequent routine treatment appointments (i.e., using a broad range of therapeutic approaches) did in fact reduce subsequent attempts in the experimental group over the 4-month follow-up period. The results are limited, however, by the brief nature of follow-up monitoring. Interestingly, of the three studies addressing more intensive follow-up as an *additive component* to treatment as usual, the two with negative results purposefully excluded high-risk patients (i.e., as defined by factors such as a history of multiple attempts, active psychiatric treatment or diagnosis, or comorbid problems). The one study that included, and actually targeted, high-risk cases was by Welu (1977). The pattern of results might well suggest that more intensive outpatient treatment, irrespective of approach, is most appropriate and effective for those identified as high risk as indicated by psychiatric diagnosis, a history of multiple attempts, or comorbidity.

Of the long-term treatment studies, one evaluated the efficacy of dialectical behavior therapy (DBT; Linehan, Armstrong, Suarez, Allmon, & Heard, 1991) and the other the role of more *intensive long-term* follow-up care cutting across multiple therapeutic approaches, rather than a specific therapy model (Allard, Marshall, & Plante, 1992). In summary, of the total of 14 studies addressing treatment outcome, only 8 actually evaluated the efficacy of a specific therapy.

As mentioned previously, for the studies evaluating the efficacy of brief cognitive-behavioral approaches, integrating a *core* problem-solving component, results were fairly uniform with 7 of 10 rendering positive findings. Although differences were not found with respect to suicide attempts, results indicated reductions in suicidal ideation (Joiner et al., 1998b; Liberman & Eckman, 1981; Salkovkis, Atha, & Storer, 1990) and related symptomatology such as depression (Lerner & Clum, 1990; Liberman & Eckman, 1981; Salkovkis et al., 1990), hopelessness (Lerner & Clum, 1990; Patsiokas & Clum, 1985), and loneliness (Lerner & Clum, 1990) over follow-up periods ranging from 3 months to 1 year. Only a single study (McLeavey, Daly, Ludgate, & Murray, 1994) found a reduction in suicide attempts at 12 months posttreatment. The findings are, however, compromised by a number of methodological problems including a small sample size, failure to include a broad range of attempters, and, most important, the purposeful exclusion of high-risk patients. Interestingly, several of these short-term treatment studies specifically targeted the highest-risk cases, that is, multiple attempters. (Joiner et al., 1998b; Liberman & Eckman, 1981; Rudd, Joiner, & Rahab, 1996; Salkovkis et al., 1990). In addition, the study by Salkovkis et al. (1990) found a reduction in attempts at 6 months, but the findings were not maintained over the full year of follow-up.

The three studies rendering negative findings found no reductions in suicide attempts during 9- to 12-month follow-up periods (Gibbons et al., 1978; Hawton et al., 1987; van der Sande et al., 1997). As with a number of the other studies, all excluded those at highest risk for subsequent attempts. Additional problems for these studies, which raise questions about the findings, included poorly defined treatments that did not appear to be applied in a uniform manner. Actually, in the study by Hawton et al. (1987), less than 50% of the experimental group actually completed treatment, but, nonetheless, subsequent comparisons included *nonattenders* and *dropouts*, seriously confounding the results. Those who did not successfully complete the treatment would, more than likely, appear comparable to the controls, rendering interpretation of the results problematic, if not impossible. Similarly, in the study by van der Sande et al. (1997), an intent-to-treat analysis was conducted, with no information provided about the number of those in the experimental group that actually completed treatment or how treatment completion was defined. It is entirely possible that many of those in the experimental group simply did not follow through with treatment, a possibility bolstered by high attrition rates.

In terms of long-term treatment, the results were mixed. Linehan et al. (1991) demonstrated the efficacy of DBT in reducing subsequent attempts, hospital days, and improving treatment compliance over a year follow-up period. No differences were found between DBT and treatment as usual, however, with respect to depression, hopelessness, suicidal ideation, or reasons for living. Her results, along with those of Rudd, Rajab, et al. (1996), suggest that outpatient treatment of high-risk suicidal patients is not only safe but can be effective when acute hospitalization is available. In contrast, Allard et al. (1992) did not find a reduction in subsequent attempts at 24 months but used a mixture of therapeutic approaches, with some questions as to the nature of the specific treatment provided as well as methodological concerns about uniformity of application. Essentially, there were questions as to whether or not all subjects received a uniform intervention and treatment that could be reasonably evaluated, rendering interpretation of findings questionable.

Implications for Clinical Practice

As with the intervention studies reviewed, available treatment outcome results allow for only a few conclusions. They are, nonetheless, important and provide an emerging scientific foundation to the treatment of suicidality. The following conclusions have adequate support in the existing literature:

1. Intensive, longer-term treatment following an attempt is most appropriate and effective for those identified as high risk as indicated by multiple attempts, psychiatric history, and diagnostic comorbidity.
2. Short-term CBT, integrating problem-solving training as a *core inter-*

vention, is effective at reducing suicidal ideation, depression, and hopelessness over periods of up to 1 year. Such brief approaches do not appear effective at reducing attempts over enduring time frames.

3. Reducing suicide attempts requires longer-term treatment and treatment modalities targeting specific skill deficits such as emotion regulation, poor distress tolerance (i.e., impulsivity), anger management, and interpersonal assertiveness, as well as other enduring problems such as interpersonal relationships and self-image disturbance (i.e., personality disorders).

4. High-risk suicidal patients can be safely and effectively treated on an outpatient basis if acute hospitalization is available and accessible.

The Therapeutic Relationship in Treating Suicidality: Attachment, Hope, and Survival

There is a wealth of evidence that the therapeutic relationship and alliance are key variables in predicting successful outcomes across different types of treatments (e.g., Gaston, Thompson, Gallagher, Cournoyer, & Gagon, 1998). The importance of the therapeutic relationship in psychotherapeutic work with suicidal patients cannot be overstated. In fact, because of issues raised in this and later chapters (e.g., the inherent challenges of assessing and treating suicidality, fear of losing patients, anxiety related to malpractice liability, and time constraints) the need for a solid relationship and strong alliance may be particularly germane to successful clinical work with suicidal patients (Jobes & Maltsberger, 1995). Actually, Bongar, Peterson, Harris, and Aissis (1989) stressed that the quality of the therapeutic alliance is one of the most significant factors in assessing risk and predicting treatment outcome in suicidality. Similarly, Simon (1988), Maltsberger (1986), London (1986), and Shneidman (1981, 1984) all have emphasized that a solid therapeutic relationship is *essential* to the successful treatment of suicidality. Without it, it is simply unlikely that the patient would even continue in treatment, not to mention invest the energy and time necessary for difficult and productive change.

Motto (1979) coined the term "active relatedness" to apply to those behaviors on the part of the clinician that facilitate attachment and alliance (e.g., emergency availability, scheduling more frequent and longer appointments, and promptness in returning phone calls). Shneidman (1981, 1984) noted that it is, often, necessary for the clinician to foster dependency in order to facilitate the initial attachment essential for ongoing care, although he encouraged caution when longer-term treatment is involved, particularly with severely personality disordered patients. Similarly, Linehan (1993) noted that "a strong, positive relationship with a suicidal patient is absolutely essential" (p. 514) for successful treatment, stating that "validation forms the core of DBT" (p. 221). She identified three strategies for addressing relationship issues in psychotherapy: relationship acceptance, relationship problem solving, and relationship generalization. Relationship acceptance simply refers to *accepting* the patient *as is*, relationship problem solving refers to active discussion of identified problems with the therapeutic relationship during therapy sessions and in outside consultation (i.e., for the clinician), and relationship generalization refers to efforts on the part of the patient to *generalize* relationship gains outside of the therapy context.

The challenges of working with such patients may elicit nontherapeutic reactions in the clinician (e.g., fear, malice, aversion, "empathic dread," hate, anxiety, and worry) which may lead to an avoidant or fear-based form of treatment that is not in the patient's best interest. Actually, Maltsberger and Buie (1974, 1989) have referred to the emergence of *countertransference hate* in the treatment of suicidal patients as a particularly destructive and malignant reaction, one that if unchecked can lead to behaviors that adversely affect the emotional well-being of the patient, not to mention the clinician. Linehan (1993) talked about the *therapy interfering behaviors of the therapist*, including a broad range of behaviors (e.g., being late for appointments, ending sessions early, eating or drinking during sessions, taking telephone calls or pages during sessions, and falling asleep). From a purely CBT perspective, Burns and Auerbach (1996) talked about the role of *therapeutic empathy* and, at times, the lack of it in psychotherapy. They offer an *empathy training program* to address the problem, integrating what are referred to as listening skills (i.e., the disarming technique, thought empathy, feeling empathy, and inquiry) and self-expression skills (i.e., "I feel" statements, stroking).

Fortunately, training and knowledge in clinical suicidology can lead to relative openness and clinical confidence so that the clinician can build a healing relationship through empathic fortitude, consistency, honesty, and perseverance. Critically, through such a relationship, suicidal patients can experience tangible relief from their sense of profound despair and realize a potentially life-saving connection in the midst of their inner experience of being abjectly alone (Jobes & Maltsberger, 1995). Being able to establish such a relationship, maintain it, monitor it, and periodically evaluate it with a critical eye is the bedrock of psychotherapy for suicidality.

Implications for Clinical Practice

In short, we draw several conclusions. First, the therapeutic relationship is vital to effective treatment of suicidality. The best techniques applied without error at precisely the right time are of limited, if any, value when an adequate therapeutic relationship and treatment alliance does not exist. In working with suicidal patients, the nature of the therapeutic relationship will take the form of prominent attachment, at least initially. Separation is an issue addressed later in the treatment process. In treating suicidality, it is often the quality of this attachment that determines subsequent treatment success. It is the trust inherent in the therapeutic relationship that allows the patient to take the necessary risks, do things differently, reach out during periods of acute and excruciating vulnerability, and experiment with new skills, all essential for progress and recovery. At times, the attachment in therapy will be the *one thing* patients can count on, the thing that gives them hope and translates to survival during particularly trying moments and early crises.

A second conclusion is that specific steps can be taken to develop, enhance, evaluate, and maintain this relationship. If the therapeutic relationship is an identifiable treatment target, then interventions can be used purposefully and strategically to facilitate, enhance, monitor, and evaluate it. A third and final conclusion is that the therapeutic relationship serves multiple purposes in treating suicidality; it is essentially a mechanism or vehicle for support, modeling, acceptance, trust, teaching, attachment, and ultimately separation and growth. In essence, it is the *vehicle of change*, particularly for those presenting with chronic suicidality and multiple attempts. For the vast majority of multiple attempters, interpersonal issues are at the core of their suicidality.

Unanswered Questions: The Challenge Awaits Us

Across the three categories mentioned earlier, intervention studies, short-term treatment, and long-term treatment, two of the studies were uninterpretable due to serious methodological flaws. Another four studies rendered questionable findings secondary to methodological problems. Of the 22 original studies, 16 provided interpretable results using sound designs. As indicated, those findings are relatively limited in terms of implications for day-to-day treatment and ongoing clinical management of suicidality.

As stated earlier in this chapter, we can answer only a few of the most fundamental questions raised about the treatment of suicidality. There appears to be an emerging trend for the efficacy of CBT, both over the short and long term. It appears that CBT, integrating problem solving as a *core intervention,* is effective at reducing suicidal ideation and related symptoms over the short term. Reducing attempts appears to require longer-term and more intensive treatment, with a specific focus on skill deficits and related personality dysfunction. Clearly, the most difficult scientific work is ahead of us. Of the questions posed earlier, all are yet to be answered in any definitive manner. Nonetheless, CBT does appear to offer considerable promise in the psychotherapeutic treatment of suicidality. More than likely, this is a function of its specific focus on both cognitive and related skill deficits. Building on this empirical foundation, Chapter 2 provides a CBT model of suicidality, one that will help the practicing clinician accomplish multiple tasks critical to effective and efficient treatment.

2

A Cognitive-Behavioral Model of Suicidality

Existing Theoretical Models of Suicidal Behavior: A Brief Overview

The study of suicide and suicidal behavior has been approached from varied and often competing theoretical and empirical models. There has been limited productive interaction around questions of empirical findings that have clinical relevance and how to apply them and, conversely, those clinical observations that warrant detailed empirical study and how to actually operationalize them in day-to-day practice. We hope that Chapter 1 has clarified this debate, at least with respect to the empirical findings that actually have implications for clinical practice.

For the most part, researchers have focused on theory and practicing clinicians have been forced to use approaches, over both the short and long term, with little if any empirical support for their efficacy. Amazingly, the most common treatment intervention for suicidality—hospitalization—continues without a single controlled study regarding its efficacy, differential effect, or actual need based on severity or complexity of diagnostic presentation (Linehan, 1997). With only a handful of controlled studies, compromised for the most part by small samples among a host of other serious methodological problems previously summarized, a solid empirical base simply does not exist in the suicidality treatment literature (e.g., Chowdury et al., 1973; Gibbons et al., 1978; Hawton et al., 1981; Hawton et al., 1987; Lerner & Clum, 1990; Liberman & Eckman, 1981; Linehan, 1993; Linehan et al., 1991; McLeavey,

Daly, Ludgate, & Murray, 1994; Motto, 1976; Patsiokas & Clum, 1985; Salkovkis et al., 1990; Rudd, Rajab, et al., 1996; van der Sande et al., 1997).

To date, a broad range of theories have driven both clinical practice and empirical studies. Included among the most frequently cited theoretical approaches to suicidality are the following: (1) epidemiological (e.g., Dublin, 1963), (2) philosophical (e.g., Battin, 1982), (3) sociocultural (e.g., Hendin, 1964), (4) sociological (Durkheim, 1897/1951), (5) psychiatric (e.g., Kraeplin, 1883/1915), (6) psychodynamic (e.g., Freud, 1917/1957), (7) psychological (e.g., Shneidman, 1985), and (8) biological (e.g., Bunney & Fawcett, 1965). Naturally, each approach has emphasized a distinctive feature, aspect, or characteristic of suicide and suicidal behavior, frequently to the purposeful exclusion of others.

Epidemiological approaches have focused on demographic characteristics, philosophical theorists have attempted to answer difficult questions the nature and purpose of life, and sociocultural and sociological researchers have emphasized the critical role played by societal and cultural variables. Similarly, psychiatric, psychodynamic, psychological, and biological researchers have stressed the importance of mental illness, unconscious conflicts and emotional processes, psychological pain and unmet psychological needs, and biochemical imbalances, respectively. Only recently has a concerted effort been made toward theoretical integration in suicidology (Maris, Berman, Maltsberger, & Yufit, 1992). Despite a rich and broad research literature, the narrow and exclusive focus of most theoretical approaches has greatly limited their clinical and practical utility. Accordingly, practitioners often struggle to apply research findings in a meaningful way in their daily clinical work with suicidal patients, opting instead to use multiple theoretical paradigms to understand, explain, and ultimately treat different aspects of a single patient's presentation. This occurs despite the strong possibility of violating stated fundamental assumptions and principles on which the theoretical approaches were developed and based.

Empirically derived models have also tended to be restrictive and somewhat exclusionary in focus. Although not specific to suicidality, a number of models have been explored and validated for depression, the most extreme manifestation of which incorporates a suicidal component. Researchers have explored the role of a broad range of variables in depression, including attributional style (e.g., Abramson, Metalsky, & Alloy, 1989), hopelessness (Beck, Brown, Berchick, Stewart, & Steer, 1990), problem solving (Nezu, Nezu, & Perri, 1989), interpersonal relationships and social reinforcement (e.g., Lewinsohn, 1975), and cognitive rigidity and distortion (e.g., Beck, Rush, Shaw, & Emery, 1979). The majority of the models proposed that are specific to suicide and suicidal behavior are, essentially, variations of the diathesis–stress–hopelessness paradigm, well articulated by Schotte and Clum (1982, 1987). A range of variables have been identified as underlying diatheses or vulnerabilities triggered by stress, both acute and chronic. Among the most frequently cited diatheses are dysfunctional assumptions (Beck, Steer, & Brown, 1993; Bonner & Rich, 1987; Ellis & Ratliff, 1986; Ranieri, Steer, Lavrence, Rissmiller, Piper, & Beck, 1987), cognitive distortions (Prezant & Neimeyer, 1988), interpersonal problem-solving deficits (Linehan, Camper, Chiles, Strosahl, & Shearin, 1987; Orbach, Rosenheim, & Harry, 1987; Rotheram-Borus, Trautman, Dopkins, & Shrout, 1990; Rudd, Rajab, & Dahm, 1994; Schotte & Clum, 1982, 1987), and cognitive rigidity (Neuringer, 1968; Neuringer & Lettieri, 1971).

Static and Dynamic Variables Predicting Suicidality

A host of other variables have been found to have value in predicting suicidal ideation, attempts (i.e., both single and multiple), and ultimately completions at a univariate level. It is perhaps easiest to summarize the existing literature by differentiating between static variables (i.e., those that are descriptive and enduring in nature) and dynamic variables (those that are more acute and alterable, varying in their meaning to the patient, intensity, and occurrence over time). Included among the static variables are the following: (1) age (i.e., escalation of risk with age particularly over age 45) (Buda & Tsuang, 1990; Patterson, Dohn, Bird, & Patterson, 1983), (2) sex (i.e., greater risk for males relative to females) (Berman & Jobes, 1991, Garrison, 1992), (3) previous psychiatric diagnosis (Axis I or II) (Fawcett et al., 1990; Murphy & Wetzel, 1990; Tanney, 1992), (4) previous history of suicidal behavior (Rudd, Joiner, & Rajab, 1996), (5) a history of suicide or suicidal behavior in the family (Roy, 1992), and (6) a history of abuse (i.e., sexual, physical, and emotional), familial violence, or punitive parenting (e.g., Linehan, 1993).

Included among those variables that are predominantly acute in nature, but a few of which are chronic or recurrent, varying over time in terms of intensity, meaning to the patient, and the degree to which they are potentially debilitating, are the following: (1) identifiable stressors with a particular focus on losses (i.e., loss of job, financial status, relationships, sense of identity, and physical or cognitive ability) (e.g., Hatton, Valente, & Rink, 1977; Yufit & Bongar, 1992) and health problems (DiBianco, 1979; Yufit & Bongar, 1992); (2) a current Axis I psychiatric diagnosis with a focus on affective disorders, substance abuse, and schizophrenia, as well as Axis I comorbidity (Fawcett et al., 1990; Murphy & Wetzel, 1990; Rudd, Dahm, & Rajab, 1993; Tanney, 1992); (3) a current Axis II diagnosis, particularly a diagnosis of borderline personality disorder (e.g., Linehan, 1993; Rudd, Joiner, & Rajab, 1996); (4) current markers of emotional dysphoria or symptom severity including anger, depression, hopelessness, helplessness, guilt, anxiety/panic, anhedonia, insomnia, and diminished attention-concentration (e.g., Fawcett et al., 1990;

Rudd, Joiner, & Rajab, 1996; Weissman, Fox, & Klerman, 1973); (5) cognitive rigidity and indications of poor problem solving or impaired coping (Patsiokas, Clum, & Luscomb, 1979; Rudd et al., 1994; Schotte & Clum, 1982, 1987); (6) social isolation and limited social support (e.g., Rudd, 1993); (7) impulse control problems such as active substance abuse, aggressive behavior, risk taking, or sexual acting out (e.g., Brown, Markku, Linnoila, & Goodwin, 1992); and (8) active suicidal thinking and associated behaviors (e.g., Clark & Fawcett, 1992).

Regardless of approach or theoretical orientation, findings are highly consistent with respect to the crucial role of hopelessness in both depression and suicidality. Findings are relatively uniform with respect to ideation, attempts, and completions in clinical samples, confirming the mediational role of hopelessness (Beck, Brown, Berchick, Stewart, & Steer, 1990; Beck, Kovacs, & Weissman, 1975; Rudd, Joiner, & Rajab, 1996). Although results are less clear in nonclinical samples and with adolescents, this chapter focuses specifically on suicidality in adults, an area in which there is little room for debate about the importance of hopelessness, its almost uniform presence, and considerable predictive power.

Application of Theory and Empirical Findings in Treatment: The Problem of Limited Clinical Relevance

The narrow focus of theoretical and empirically derived models is understandable and entirely warranted. Good science is characterized by specificity in theory, investigation, and application. Theoretical discussions and arguments and empirical findings to date all have greatly benefited the clinician setting in the office, one on one with the suicidal patient. However, one of the primary difficulties for practitioners attempting to employ these models in treatment is their *limited clinical relevance*. They are often difficult to apply in individual treatment cases given subtle but important distinctions and nuances presented by individual patients. Most clinicians agree that suicidal patients are the most diagnostically complex and therapeutically challenging patients they see (e.g., Pope & Tabachnick, 1993), which is consistent with the complexity of suicidality itself, a problem inarguably the result of a complex web of factors with precise interrelationships varying from individual to individual. This is true despite consistency in empirical studies regarding the roles of such variables as life stress, problem solving, hopelessness, and emotion regulation (Rudd, 2000).

As a result, the nature of treatment provided varies somewhat and is not uniform across all the cases of suicidality that any one clinician treats. Undeniably, different variables have different meanings and varying levels of importance for different cases in clinical practice. At times, practitioners are faced with what appears to be a disparate group of predictor variables and correlates of suicidality that are not woven together in a coherent and clinically accessible model that can be applied with some uniformity *across* different cases.

To date, efforts to apply the existing theoretical and empirical literature on suicidology in clinical settings has resulted in several identifiable and consistent problems. First, there is the narrow conceptual focus, discussed earlier, resulting in cumbersome and imprecise application both within and across individual cases. Although the narrow focus of many theoretical models allows for considerable depth and detail in explaining *specific aspects* of suicidality, the models tend to be paradoxically simplistic when applied clinically. As a result, they do not provide a meaningful and comprehensive explanatory framework for patients, despite affording the clinician a general conceptual guide for treatment. It is difficult to account for the individual differences both between and within patients and to model them in a precise and meaningful way using the majority of the conceptualizations currently available. It is not uncommon for practitioners to employ multiple paradigms to explain and address different aspects of a single patient's presentation (e.g., Axis I and II comorbidity). For example, hopelessness might be approached from a cognitive perspective, employing standard techniques and interventions. Conversely, prominent depressive symptoms might be explained biologically, with medication as the primary treatment intervention. Problems potentially consistent with an Axis II component such as persistent emotional dysphoria, a chronic desire to die, and interpersonal conflict might be explained and treated from a psychodynamic point of view. The net result is an unusual mixture of potentially conflictual paradigms, with little acknowledgment of underlying inconsistency in theory, fundamental assumptions, and the resultant impact on treatment process, duration, or outcome.

A second problem is the potential confusion and lack of clarity for the patient as to what exactly is being targeted in treatment, how it is explained, and how it is to be ameliorated. Mixing and matching paradigms and problems can result in considerable difficulty in communicating in a coherent and consistent fashion with patients. Third, as hinted at previously, many models lack specificity in terms of identifiable treatment targets across *all* domains of human functioning, including cognitive, biological, emotional, behavioral, and interpersonal (i.e., situational and environmental). Rather, there has been a tendency, consistent with the narrow focus of some approaches, to target isolated although critical variables. This tendency results in a fourth problem: difficulty in comprehensive treatment outcome monitoring and a corresponding lack of clarity for patients as to what actually denotes treatment success or progress. If the treatment approach is exclusionary and narrow in focus, progress in one domain can simply go unnoticed, regardless of how significant. Similarly, the use of multiple paradigms can result in broad categorizations and related confusion that does not lend itself to specific treatment targets.

In the end, somewhat of a compromise is needed; an inclusive conceptual framework that allows for direct clinical application of empirical findings across *specific* areas of functioning (i.e., cognitive, emotional, biological, behavioral, and interpersonal). Such a model would address the broad range of factors empirically validated as relevant, incorporating Axis I and II diagnostic components. As has been discussed by others, cognitive theory and therapy offers a unique foundation for such integrative efforts (Alford & Beck, 1997). There are consistencies both in theory and empirical findings that provide the necessary foundation for an integrative cognitive-behavioral model of suicidality, one that is flexible enough for application in day-to-day clinical practice and rigorous enough for experimental investigation. As reviewed in Chapter 1, an impressive trend is emerging regarding the efficacy of CBT for the treatment of suicidality, over both the short and long term. In terms of treatment outcome studies, it is simply the only observable trend in a limited database.

Basic Assumptions of Cognitive Theory and Therapy: Implications for Suicidality

In applying cognitive theory to the psychopathology of suicidality and subsequent psychotherapy, it is critical to be aware of the fundamental assumptions that are operative. Essentially, the inherent assumptions guide the nature of the clinical work itself, determining treatment content, the nature of its application and course followed, and subsequent therapeutic process, as well as the definition and conceptualization of treatment outcome and related monitoring. Clark (1995) summarized the fundamental assumptions of cognitive therapy as follows: (1) individuals actively participate in the construction of their reality, (2) cognitive therapy is a mediational theory, (3) cognition is knowable and accessible, (4) cognitive change is central to the human change process, and finally (5) cognitive therapy adopts a present time frame. These assumptions are relatively broad in nature but, nonetheless, provide a conceptual framework for cognitive theory and its application to suicidality.

In their statement of a formal cognitive theory, Alford and Beck (1997) went far beyond the fundamental assumptions summarized by Clark (1995). They offered considerable detail with the following 10 axioms:

1. The central pathway to psychological functioning or adaptation consists of the meaning-making structures of cognition, termed *schemas*. [. . .]
2. The function of *meaning assignment* (at both automatic and deliberate levels) is to control the various psychological systems (e.g., behavioral, emotional, attentional, and memory). [. . .]
3. The influences between cognitive systems and other systems are interactive.

4. Each category of meaning has implications that are translated into specific patterns of emotion, attention, memory, and behavior. This is termed *cognitive content specificity*.

5. Although meanings are constructed by the person, rather than being preexisting components of reality, they are correct or incorrect in relation to a given context or goal. When *cognitive distortions* or *bias* occurs, meanings are dysfunctional or maladaptive. Cognitive distortions include errors in cognitive content (meaning), cognitive processing (meaning elaboration), or both.

6. Individuals are predisposed to specific faulty cognitive constructions (cognitive distortions). These predispositions to specific distortions are termed *cognitive vulnerabilities*. Specific cognitive vulnerabilities predispose persons to specific syndromes; cognitive specificity and cognitive vulnerability are interrelated.

7. Psychopathology results from maladaptive meanings constructed regarding the self, the environmental context (experience), and the future (goals), which together are termed the *cognitive triad*. Each clinical syndrome has characteristic maladaptive meanings associated with the components of the cognitive triad. [. . .]

8. There are two levels of meaning: (a) the objective or *public meaning* of an event, which may have few significant implications for an individual; and (b) the *personal or private meaning*. The personal meaning, unlike the public one, includes implications, significance, or generalizations drawn from occurrence of the event. [. . .]

9. There are three levels of cognition: (a) the preconscious, unintentional, *automatic* level ("automatic thoughts"); (b) the conscious level; and (c) the metacognitive level, which includes "realistic" or "rational" (adaptive) responses. These serve useful functions, but the conscious levels are of primary interest for clinical improvement in psychotherapy. [. . .]

10. Schemas evolved to facilitate adaptation of the person to the environment, and are in this sense *telenomic* structures. Thus, a given psychological state (constituted by the activation of systems) is neither adaptive nor maladaptive in itself, but only in relation to or in the context of the larger social and physical environment in which the person resides. (pp. 15–17; emphasis in original)

As evidenced by the fundamental assumptions offered by Clark (1995) and the axioms detailed by Alford and Beck (1997), application of cognitive theory and therapy to suicidality requires us to be detailed and specific in our thinking and approach.

Available empirical findings in suicidology are well suited to a cognitive-behavioral theoretical framework. Although cognitive theory and therapy purports that the *central pathway to psychological functioning* is cognition (i.e., meaning-making structures identified as schemas), the approach is mediational in nature, consistent with an integrative and interactional model

essential to suicidality. As noted in axiom 3, the relationship between the cognitive and other systems (e.g., biological/physiological and emotional, behavioral) is interactive. At the most fundamental level, the cognitive-behavioral
model asserts reciprocal determinism between the environment and person
(e.g., Bandura, 1986). An individual does not live in isolation but in a dynamic
context, with reciprocal influence, interaction, and interdependent outcome
across the previously noted domains (i.e., cognitive, emotional, behavioral,
biological/physiological, and interpersonal). Some of the more consistent and
clinically relevant empirical findings can easily be woven into a meaningful
explanatory model using this framework.

The 10 axioms of cognitive theory offered by Alford and Beck (1997)
translate into a number of identifiable *fundamental assumptions* when applied
to suicidality and related psychotherapeutic treatment. They are as follows:

1. The central pathway for suicidality is cognition (i.e., the *private* meaning assigned by the individual). Suicidality is secondary to maladaptive meaning
constructed and assigned regarding the self, the environmental context, and the
future (i.e., the cognitive triad, along with related conditional assumptions/rules
and compensatory strategies, referred to as the *suicidal belief system*).

2. The relationship between the *suicidal belief system* (i.e., cognitive
triad specific to the *suicidal mode* discussed later) and the other psychological (e.g., behavioral, emotional, attentional, and memory) and biological/
physiological systems is interactive and interdependent.

3. The *suicidal belief system* will vary from individual to individual, depending on the content and context of the various psychological systems (i.e.,
cognitive content specificity). Nonetheless, there will be some uniformity in
terms of identified *categories* (i.e., helplessness, unlovability, and poor distress tolerance; all discussed in more detail later), all tinged by a pervasive
sense of hopelessness.

4. Individuals are predisposed to suicidality as a function of cognitive
vulnerabilities, or *faulty cognitive constructions,* which covary with specific
syndromes. Accordingly, different cognitive vulnerabilities are consistent with
different syndromes and patterns of comorbidity, both Axis I and II.

5. Suicidality and the *suicidal belief system* reside at three distinct levels,
the preconscious or automatic level, the conscious level, and the metacognitive (i.e., unconscious) level, with the conscious levels most amenable to
psychotherapeutic change. The structural content of the suicidal belief system,
at all three levels, is contained within the *suicidal mode*, a concept discussed
in more detail later.

The assumptions summarized offer a foundation from which to articulate
a conceptual model to treat all aspects of the suicidal patient, cutting across
multiple domains and incorporating a broad range of empirical work but also

allowing flexibility to address the considerable individual differences encountered in clinical settings. In addition, the assumptions summarized provide a solid theoretical foundation for the CBT models used in the treatment outcome studies reviewed in Chapter 1 (this volume), facilitating interpretation regarding the nature and duration of treatment effect.

The Essential Requirements for a Cognitive-Behavioral Model of Suicidality: Integrating Empirical Findings and Ensuring Clinical Relevance

Based on the theoretical framework discussed so far and the assumptions summarized earlier, a CBT model of suicidality needs to incorporate, or account for, the major and most consistent empirical findings in the field. In addition, to have clinical relevance, it needs to be understandable, flexible, and modifiable for application in day-to-day clinical settings. In short, the following 10 requirements are essential to a comprehensive and clinically relevant CBT model of suicidality:

1. The model needs to address those variables (across all domains of functioning including cognitive, affective, behavioral, motivational) in a fashion unique to the patient's presentation and in a manner understandable to the patient. In other words, the model will serve as a parsimonious explanatory *map* of the presenting psychopathology. It needs to account for and communicate to both therapist and patient the symptomatic presentation, relevant developmental history and trauma, prominent maladaptive personality traits, identifiable stressors, and behavioral responses in an integrative, rather than isolated, fashion. Consistent with the notion of a *treatment map*, it needs to explain for the therapist and patient how the patient got from point *A* (nonsuicidal) to point *B* (suicidal) and how he or she gets to point *C* (recovery).

2. The model needs to communicate the transient, time-limited nature of suicidal crises, even for those exhibiting recurrent and chronic suicidal behavior. By definition, crises are self-limiting. Even those individuals who present with chronic suicidality are at imminent risk for only limited periods, consistent with Litman's (1990) idea of the *suicide zone*.

3. The model needs to identify individual vulnerabilities that predispose to multiple suicidal crises or recurrent behavior, acknowledging the importance of Axis I and II diagnoses, and related comorbidity, along with developmental trauma and personal history.

4. The model needs to provide a means of distinguishing between suicidal, self-destructive, and self-mutilatory behaviors, accounting for distinct differences in the three across each domain of functioning.

5. The model needs to integrate the role of triggering events, accounting for acute and chronic stressors as well as personality disturbance. In particular, the model needs to acknowledge the potentially significant role of *internal* triggers (i.e., thoughts, images, feelings, and physical sensations).

6. The model needs to integrate the importance of emotion regulation, emotional dysphoria, and distress tolerance in the suicidal process.

7. The model needs to address the importance of interpersonal factors and social reinforcement in maintaining the behavior or facilitating recovery.

8. The model needs to provide sufficient explanatory detail so as to translate into a specific treatment plan, that is, identifiable treatment targets across all domains of functioning.

9. The model needs to facilitate self-monitoring and self-awareness, providing flexibility in explaining day-to-day functioning. This can only be accomplished if the model is straightforward and easy to understand, relying on well-defined theoretical constructs.

10. The model needs to account for the process of change in suicidality over time, not just in terms of presenting symptoms. It needs to incorporate the idea of skill acquisition, development, and refinement (i.e., personality change). It needs to reflect this change at multiple levels and across multiple domains of functioning.

The Suicidal Mode as a Cognitive-Behavioral Model of Suicidality: An Elaboration and Specific Application of Beck's Theory of Modes and Psychopathology

Beck (1996) recently offered a refinement of his original cognitive therapy model in response to a growing body of empirical studies and theoretical discourse that highlighted a number of shortcomings in efforts to explain more complex theoretical constructs and related interactions and to experimentally validate them (e.g., Haaga, Dyck, & Ernst, 1991). The model is consistent with the axioms noted previously and builds on the concept of schemas and simple linear schema processing in a number of important ways. The theory is built around the concept of the *mode*, the structural or organizational unit that contains schemas. Beck (1996) has defined modes as "specific suborganizations within the personality organization [that] incorporate the relevant components of the basic systems of personality: cognitive (information processing), affective, behavioral, and motivational" (p. 4). He went on to note that, consistent with the original theory, each system is composed of structures identified as schemas (e.g., affective schemas, cognitive schemas, behavioral schemas, and motivational schemas). Beck has integrated the physiological system as separate but noted its unique and significant contribution to the overall functioning of the mode. Of particular importance to the concept of the mode is the previously noted issue of reciprocal determinism and synchrony of action. Beck (1996) has described the mode as an "integrated cognitive-affective-behavioral network that provides a synchronous response to external demands and provides a mechanism for implementing internal dictates and goals" (p. 4).

The *cognitive system* is described as involving all aspects of information processing including selection of data, attentional process (i.e., meaning assignment and meaning making), memory, and subsequent recall. Incorporated within this system is the notion of the *cognitive triad,* integrating beliefs regarding self, others, and the future. For our discussion of the *suicidal mode,* the representative cognitive triad, along with the associated conditional assumptions/rules and compensatory strategies, is referred to as the suicidal belief system. Consistent with axiom 6 (Alford & Beck, 1997), three levels of cognition are assumed, with the majority of therapeutic efforts targeting the more conscious levels. This does not negate, however, the importance of preconscious and metacognitive processing. In addition, it provides a means of integrating research and theory on implicit learning and tacit knowledge (e.g., Dowd & Courchaine, 1996).

The *affective system* produces emotional and affective experience. Beck (1996) noted the importance of the affective system, emphasizing its role in reinforcing adaptive behavior through the experience of both positive and negative affect (Beck, Emery, & Greenberg, 1985). This makes both conceptual and logical sense. He went on to state that negative affective experiences *focus the attention* of individuals on circumstances or situational contexts that are not in our best interest or serve "to diminish [us] in some way" (p. 5). As a result, a negative valence is created for that event, situation, or experience, increasing sensitivity of the mode to being triggered or activated in the future under comparable circumstances. This helps explain low threshold for activation for some suicidal patients as well as generalization across similar but not entirely identical situations or circumstances. For multiple attempters, then, they would not only have a lower *activation threshold* but also a broader range of internal and external triggers.

Finally, the *motivational and behavioral systems* allow for autonomic activation or deactivation of the individual for response. Although Beck noted that the motivational and behavioral systems are, for the most part, automatic in activation, they can be consciously controlled under some conditions. The *physiological system* consists of the physiological symptomatology accompanying the mode. A *threat mode,* for example, would include autonomic arousal, along with motor and sensory system activation, which would orient the individual for action such as *fight or flight.* The synchronous and simultaneous interaction of multiple systems and potential cognitive misinterpretation during a threat mode lead to escalation and expansion of physical symptoms (e.g., perception of threat from panic symptoms such as "I'm having a heart attack"). Again, each system consists of structures or *schemas* specific to that system. Accordingly, the suicidal belief system is comprised of beliefs or schemas within each of the identified systems (i.e., affective schemas, behavioral schemas, and motivational schemas).

In addition, Beck (1996) distinguished more *primal modes* as reflexive and oriented toward survival, safety and security, adding that each of the clinical disorders can be distinguished by a specific *primal mode*. This is in contrast to *habitual* or prevailing modes representative of prominent personality traits, adaptive and maladaptive, that are a constant in the individual's life. As a means of explaining excessive reaction in clinical disorders, Beck asserts that a mode can become highly *charged*, an idea essentially consistent with the concept of a low threshold for activation or negative valence for maladaptive modes such as the suicidal mode. In contrast, *minor modes* are not highly charged, allow for higher thresholds before activation, and are under more flexible conscious control.

Beck's (1996) theory of modes and psychopathology offers a number of advantages over earlier versions of simple linear schematic processing, particularly for understanding suicidality:

1. It provides a means to explain specific Axis I disorders as the result of maladaptive activation, and heightened sensitivity, of primal modes.
2. Personality disorders are viewed as dysfunctional modes that are in operation the majority of the time or, conversely, have a low threshold for activation and are triggered by a wider array of stimuli. This is consistent with findings that note different typologies for ideators, those making single attempts, multiple attempters, and those completing suicide (e.g., Orbach, 1997; Rudd, Joiner, & Rajab, 1996).
3. The cognitive *structures* comprising modes are consistent with previous cognitive conceptualizations that incorporate the cognitive triad, associated core beliefs, conditional rules/assumptions, and compensatory strategies, all tinged by hopelessness (e.g., Beck, 1996). Accordingly, the resultant conceptualizations make sense and represent a refinement over earlier efforts, bolstered by the integration of empirical findings.
4. The construct of mode provides a means to understand the diversity of symptoms experienced and diagnostic complexity and comorbidity representative of multiple systems interacting in synchrony and acknowledging the implicit complexity of phenomena such as suicidality.
5. Modes help explain observed deficits in skill acquisition, development, and refinement over time, consistent with progressive personality change and evolution in treatment (e.g., Linehan, 1993). In other

words, as individuals recover it becomes more difficult to trigger the suicidal mode (i.e., a higher threshold for activation, reduced sensitivity, and reactivity to identified triggers), facilitating modes are deactivated, and adaptive modes are created and exercised.

6. Modes explain the low threshold for triggering some suicidal crises, observed sensitization to activating stressors, and apparent habituation in the recovery process.

Defining the Suicidal Mode: Characteristics of the Various Systems

Although he mentioned a suicidal mode, Beck (1996) did not articulate the details or elaborate on the proposed mode. Before doing so, several points need to be restated and considered in more detail. First, as others have argued, it is critical for any model of suicidal behavior to clearly articulate the crucial role of *intent* (e.g., O'Carroll et al., 1996), distinguishing between suicidal, self-destructive, and self-mutilatory behaviors. Second, the model needs to account for observed variations in suicidality over time, addressing differences between those making a single attempt with no recurrence versus recurrent and chronic suicidality or what Maris (1991) coined as "suicidal careers." Third, the model needs to account for, and incorporate, the empirical findings summarized previously. Among those variables with the most importance are the somewhat mixed symptom picture often presented (e.g., considerable Axis I and II comorbidity), the clear role of stressors (both acute and chronic) in suicidality, identifiable skill deficits or diatheses, the potentially protective role of social support, and the pervasiveness of hopelessness. The concept of the mode provides a means of incorporating into an interdependent network what, at times, have been viewed and studied as disparate variables.

Table 2.1 provides a summary of the *suicidal mode*, outlining the characteristic features of each system. The next section of this chapter provides a detailed, step-by-step summary of how to complete the suicidal mode (i.e., case conceptualization) for a given patient. As indicated, the cognitive system is characterized by the suicidal belief system, incorporating the cognitive triad as well as associated conditional rules/assumptions and compensatory strategies. The core beliefs that permeate the cognitive triad fall within the two primary domains originally identified by Beck (1996), *helplessness* (e.g., "I can't do anything about my problems") and *unlovability* ("I don't deserve to live, I'm worthless"). An additional third category has also been proposed: *poor distress tolerance* ("I can't stand feeling this way anymore") (see Figure 2.1). All core beliefs voiced by a given suicidal patient will cut across these three categories or cluster in one or two categories. More often than not, though, sui-

TABLE 2.1. System Characteristics for the Suicidal Mode

System	Structural content (*Example of thought/belief*)
Cognitive	Suicidal belief system: Suicidal thoughts (*"I want to kill myself, I'm going to commit suicide."*)
	Components of cognitive triad
	Core belief categories: Unlovability, helplessness, poor distress tolerance
	• Self: inadequate, worthless, incompetent, helpless, imperfect unlovable, defective. (*"I'm worthless. Everyone else would be better off if I was dead. I can't change any of this."*)
	• Others: rejecting, abusing, abandoning, judgmental. (*"Nobody really cares about me."*)
	• Future (potential for change): hopeless. (*"Things will never change and I can't tolerate these feelings."*)
	Conditional rules/assumptions: (*"If I'm perfect then people would accept me. If I do what everyone wants then they'll have to like me."*)
	Compensatory strategies: Overcompensation, perfectionism, subjugation in relationships.
Affective	Dysphoria (mixed negative emotions): for example, sadness, anger, anxiety, guilt, depression, hurt, suspiciousness, fearfulness, tense, loneliness, embarrassment, humiliation, shame.
Behavioral (motivational)	Death-related behaviors (intent to suicide): preparatory behaviors, planning, rehearsal behaviors, attempts.
Physiological:	Arousal: autonomic, motor, sensory systems activation.

cidal patients present with core beliefs that cut across all three. Also as indicated, the future orientation is hopelessness, the primary pervasive feature of an active suicidal mode.

As discussed in more detail later, when hopelessness abates, the active intent to die simultaneously diminishes, and then the suicidal mode is no longer predominant. Other facilitating modes are active, consistent with long-standing personality disturbance and related self-destructive, self-defeating, and/or self-mutilatory behaviors. Clearly, individuals can shift in and out of the suicidal mode with great frequency and for variable periods. As mentioned earlier, it is easier to *trigger* the suicidal mode for those evidencing chronic

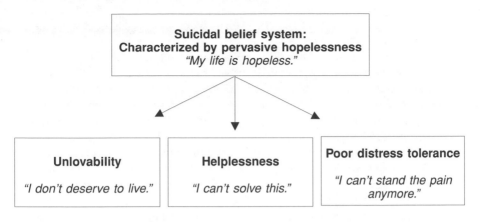

FIGURE 2.1. Core belief categories of the suicidal belief system.

suicidality. That is, they have lower activation thresholds and are hypersensitive to a wider array of stimuli.

The affective system is distinguished by emotional dysphoria, that is, a *mixture* of negative emotions. This is in contrast to the sadness characteristic of depression. Empirical findings regarding the often mixed symptom picture present dysphoria as including feelings of sadness, anxiety, anger, guilt, shame, humiliation, among a host of potential others. The behavioral (and motivational) impulse is to die, indicative of clear intent to commit suicide regardless of any subsequent outcome (e.g., a suicide attempt with injuries or no injuries). Questionable intent is manifest by variations in the behavioral impulse. For example, the desire for revenge, punishment of a significant other, or the relief of tension, agitation, or pain without the desire to die (e.g., self-destructive behavior such as illicit drug use or self-mutilatory behavior such as self-cutting, burning, or piercing) is consistent with *facilitating* modes but not an active suicidal mode.

During a period in which the suicidal mode is active, the physiological system is aroused, with autonomic, motor, and sensory system activation. As is suggested by this conceptualization, the suicidal mode is essentially *self-limiting*. That is, the physiological arousal necessary can only be maintained for limited periods, with variations likely dependent on the chronicity of the problem (i.e., single attempters vs. multiple attempters) and the complexity of the Axis I and II diagnostic picture. It is speculated that the duration of time for an active suicidal mode varies in accordance with the chronicity of the behavior. In other words, multiple attempters are likely to experience longer periods of activation of the suicidal mode in comparison to single attempters. Actually, some of our work is consistent with this possibility. We found that multiple attempters experienced suicidal crises of significantly longer duration in contrast to single attempters when an identifiable precipitant was present (Joiner & Rudd, 2000).

By definition, then, suicidal crises are acute and time limited in nature, even for those evidencing chronic disturbance and recurrent suicidal behavior. This idea is consistent with the concept of the *suicide zone* defined by Litman (1990). Essentially, the *suicide zone* represents a convergence of multiple factors (e.g., situational stress, acute emotional dysphoria, psychiatric disturbance, impaired cognitive functioning, deficient problem solving, and limited social support resources) which temporarily raise the risk of suicide significantly. In other words, the potential for suicide becomes imminent. This level of risk, however, cannot be maintained for an indeterminate period, and at some point in the future, as the contributing factors subside, risk diminishes. The notion of the *suicide zone,* although less theoretically precise, is consistent with the construct of the suicidal mode, with activation of interdependent systems that result in heightened potential for a tragic outcome over a limited amount of time.

For those evidencing chronic suicidality, the suicidal mode can be characterized by two distinctive features. First, the threshold for activation of the suicidal mode is lower for potential triggers, both internal and external. Beck (1996) used the construct of the *orienting schema* to explain activation. Essentially, orienting schemas are dependent on individual history and development. The orienting schema *assigns preliminary meaning* to the stimulus situation, activating appropriate modes. For the chronically suicidal person, the threshold for activation of the suicidal mode by orienting schema is lower in comparison to nonsuicidal individuals. Second, they can be thought of as possessing a broader range of orienting schema that serve to activate the suicidal mode in response to a greater number of situations, experiences, and environmental stimuli. In other words, suicidality is easier to trigger among multiple attempters in comparison to others. More than likely, this is the function of a gradual process of generalization from trigger to trigger. For example, to begin with, interpersonal conflict in intimate relationships only might trigger the suicidal mode. Over time, however, interpersonal conflict in general might trigger the suicidal mode, regardless of the intimacy inherent in the relationship. In other words, the stimulus generalized from *intimate* relationships to *all* relationships.

This conceptualization helps explain variations in risk over time, acknowledging that heightened risk endures for limited periods and then recurs, all depending on activation of the suicidal mode. Although *deactivated* at some point, habitual personality modes (i.e., predisposing vulnerabilities) are still operative, raising chronic or long-term risk. These modes can be thought of as *facilitating modes*, increasing the probability of future suicidal episodes. Facilitating modes can take many forms. In terms of the literature on suicidality, those modes are represented by prior Axis I and II diagnoses, earnlier suicidal behavior, developmental trauma, abuse, or neglect, and parental modeling. Essentially, the chronically suicidal person shifts between facilitating and suicidal modes recurrently over time, depending on situational context. Therefore, effective and efficient treatment has to recognize the critical and enduring role of prominent personality traits.

The suicidal mode is a conceptual model easily understood and followed by patients, incorporating relevant empirical findings into the identified systems and translating them into a framework to both articulate the content of and guide treatment. Figure 2.2 provides a graphic illustration of the proposed suicidal mode. As is evident, there is reciprocal interaction and interdependence of the various systems. Although the model as presented appears somewhat linear and sequential in nature, it is important to note the synchronous interaction of the systems described by Beck (1996) and consistent with cognitive theory and the 10 axioms offered by Alford and Beck (1997).

Predisposing vulnerabilities include those static variables previously identified as raising risk for activation of the suicidal mode, including a previous psychiatric diagnosis (Axis I and II), prior history of suicidal behavior,

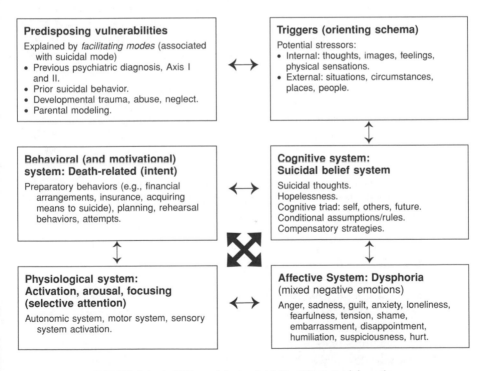

FIGURE 2.2. A CBT model of suicidality: The suicidal mode.

traumatic developmental history, and potential parental modeling. These factors are represented by the construct of the *facilitating mode*, a mode that facilitates or raises the potential for eventual activation of the suicidal mode. Again, this idea is consistent with Beck's (1996) notion of *habitual or prevailing* modes that are present most of the time, or have a low threshold for activation, and are indicative of personality psychopathology. The primary difference is that facilitating modes, although they may vary in nature from individual to individual in terms of those associated with suicidality, are thought to specifically heighten the risk for activation of the suicidal mode.

The triggers, both internal and external, are compatible with Beck's concept of the orienting schema. Depending on individual history (and predisposing vulnerabilities), there are a range of internal (thoughts, images, physical sensations, emotions) and external (stressors, situations, circumstances, people) factors that trigger the orienting schema (which assigns preliminary meaning) and *activate* the suicidal mode. This provides a conceptual role for *stressors* in the suicidal process. Once activated, the suicidal mode is fairly consistent across individual cases, with a few important distinctions. During active phases of suicidality, the cognitive system or the SBS is consumed with thoughts of death by suicide, with hopelessness pervading every component of the cognitive triad. The behavioral (and motivational) systems are characterized by an impulse to die, with related behaviors evident such as prepatory behaviors, planning, and practice or rehearsal for suicide. The affective system is characterized by dysphoria, an aversive mixture of negative emotions in varied proportions and intensities, including anger, sadness, anxiety, and guilt among others. Corresponding physiological arousal is experienced, consistent with autonomic, motor, and sensory system activation. All this occurs in synchrony and endures for a limited time, the duration of which is highly questionable. Identifying clinically relevant time frames (e.g., minutes, hours, or days) for risk is an area in considerable need of study that to date is poorly understood (Rudd & Joiner, 1998a).

The synchronous and time-limited nature of activation of the suicidal mode is perhaps best illustrated by the following journal entry by a chronically suicidal patient:

> "As I stood at the rail I began to think about climbing over and jumping. I knew if I did jump, it would kill me for sure. It's difficult to describe exactly what I felt. There was just this overwhelming pressure inside telling me if I just climbed up and jumped, all of this would be over in a few seconds. I had trouble moving back from the rail. It was as if I couldn't move—I just kept looking at the ground and thinking 'jump.' I finally made myself go inside the room. I closed the door and locked it. I sat on the bed, scared and shaking. I knew I had come very, very close to killing myself."

As evidenced, the potentially lethal nature of the situation on the balcony triggered the suicidal mode. For this patient, at the time, habitual personality modes lowered the threshold for activation. Once activated, the cognitive content was hopeless and specific, emotional dysphoria was experienced, behavior oriented toward death, and intent high. Competing compensatory modes (not facilitating) allowed for effective coping behaviors (going back inside and locking the door), assisting in deactivation and eventual recovery.

As evidenced in the example, it is important to distinguish between suicidal and nonsuicidal modes during the course of treatment, that is, those more consistent with self-destructive behaviors but not representative of clear intent to die. These modes are best described as *facilitating modes*, incorporating cognitions, affect, and behavior that heighten the risk for activation of the suicidal mode. As described in the journal entry, an individual can easily and instantaneously shift from one to another, but during acute crisis, the suicidal mode is active. As evidenced in the previous example, recovery depends on *compensatory modes* that allow for behaviors that lower risk, hasten affective recovery, and provide competing cognitions essential for cognitive restructuring. Accordingly, an accurate depiction of the patient's suicidal process would include both the active suicidal mode as well as associated facilitating modes, which are more pervasive, active more often, and comprise the bulk of treatment over the long term.

Completing the Suicidal Mode: Individual Case Conceptualization

The suicidal mode can be outlined for a patient with relative ease by answering and elaborating on six fundamental questions in stepwise fashion (see Figures 2.3 and 2.4):

1. What about the patient's history facilitates his or her suicidal behavior?
2. What triggered the suicidal crisis?
3. How does the patient think about suicide (i.e., the *suicidal belief system*)?
4. What does he or she feel during the suicidal crisis?
5. What type of arousal symptoms is the patient experiencing?
6. What suicidal behaviors have been demonstrated, planned?

Figure 2.3 provides a listing of further questions within each system that will help identify the specific structural content of the suicidal mode. As is evident, the questions provide considerable detail, expanding on the six basic questions listed previously. Figure 2.4 provides a *summary worksheet* that will help the

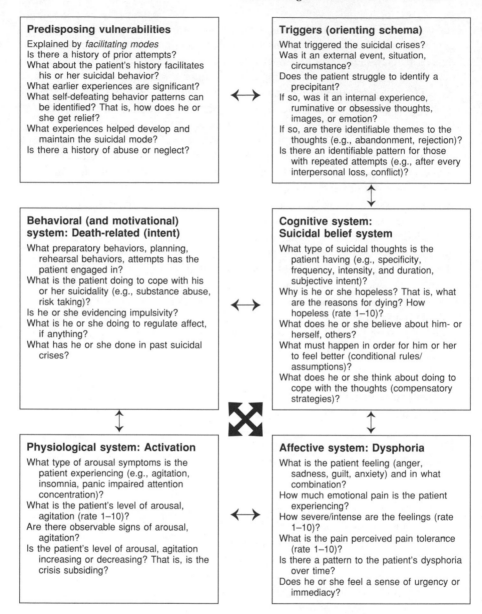

Predisposing vulnerabilities

Explained by *facilitating modes*
Is there a history of prior attempts?
What about the patient's history facilitates
    his or her suicidal behavior?
What earlier experiences are significant?
What self-defeating behavior patterns can
    be identified? That is, how does he or
    she get relief?
What experiences helped develop and
    maintain the suicidal mode?
Is there a history of abuse or neglect?

Triggers (orienting schema)

What triggered the suicidal crises?
Was it an external event, situation,
    circumstance?
Does the patient struggle to identify a
    precipitant?
If so, was it an internal experience,
    ruminative or obsessive thoughts,
    images, or emotion?
If so, are there identifiable themes to the
    thoughts (e.g., abandonment, rejection)?
Is there an identifiable pattern for those
    with repeated attempts (e.g., after every
    interpersonal loss, conflict)?

**Behavioral (and motivational)
system: Death-related (intent)**

What preparatory behaviors, planning,
    rehearsal behaviors, attempts has the
    patient engaged in?
What is the patient doing to cope with his
    or her suicidality (e.g., substance abuse,
    risk taking)?
Is he or she evidencing impulsivity?
What is he or she doing to regulate affect,
    if anything?
What has he or she done in past suicidal
    crises?

**Cognitive system:
Suicidal belief system**

What type of suicidal thoughts is the
    patient having (e.g., specificity,
    frequency, intensity, and duration,
    subjective intent)?
Why is he or she hopeless? That is, what
    are the reasons for dying? How
    hopeless (rate 1–10)?
What does he or she believe about him- or
    herself, others?
What must happen in order for him or her
    to feel better (conditional rules/
    assumptions)?
What does he or she think about doing to
    cope with the thoughts (compensatory
    strategies)?

Physiological system: Activation

What type of arousal symptoms is the
    patient experiencing (e.g., agitation,
    insomnia, panic impaired attention
    concentration)?
What is the patient's level of arousal,
    agitation (rate 1–10)?
Are there observable signs of arousal,
    agitation?
Is the patient's level of arousal, agitation
    increasing or decreasing? That is, is the
    crisis subsiding?

Affective system: Dysphoria

What is the patient feeling (anger,
    sadness, guilt, anxiety) and in what
    combination?
How much emotional pain is the patient
    experiencing?
How severe/intense are the feelings (rate
    1–10)?
What is the pain perceived pain tolerance
    (rate 1–10)?
Is there a pattern to the patient's dysphoria
    over time?
Does he or she feel a sense of urgency or
    immediacy?

FIGURE 2.3. Outlining the suicidal mode.

clinician organize all the relevant information in a fairly concise manner that can be transferred directly to the treatment plan (see Chapter 3, this volume).

As illustrated in Figures 2.3 and 2.4, completing each modal component is relatively straightforward. Predisposing vulnerabilities are captured by previous psychiatric diagnoses (Axis I and II), prior suicide attempts, early trauma (e.g., physical, emotional, sexual abuse), and a family history of suicidal behavior. To identify triggers, the clinician need simply explore any identifiable precipitants to the current and previous suicidal crises. Was it an external event, situation, or circumstance? If not, and particularly if the patient has a history of trauma, was it an internal experience, ruminative or obsessive thoughts, or images or related feelings? If so, is there a pattern or theme to the thoughts or ruminations (e.g., abandonment, harm, rejection, criticism, or abuse)? It is particularly important for the clinician to explore potential patterns or cycles for those making multiple attempts. For example, does a suicide attempt follow every interpersonal rejection? Does an attempt follow every perceived failure or insult? If patterns are identified, underlying themes can be targeted, particularly with respect to the structural content of the suicidal belief system (see Chapters 3 and 8, this volume). In all likelihood, identified interpersonal themes such as rejection or abandonment will have significant implications for the therapeutic relationship and the continuity of treatment over time (see Chapter 9, this volume).

For patients who express or acknowledge little insight into their suicidality (e.g., "It just happened, it was so fast I don't know what set it off"), use of the suicidal thought record (STR) is recommended. Figures 5.6 and 5.7 (see Chapter 5) provide examples of the STR, a simple self-monitoring instrument specific to suicidality. The STR is a straightforward elaboration of the Dysfunctional Thought Record originally developed by Beck et al. (1979) and since modified considerably for use with a broad range of clinical problems (e.g., Beck, 1995). As evidenced, the STR provides a structured means of helping the patient identify the component parts of the suicidal mode, including triggers (both internal and external) and associated suicidal thoughts and beliefs (i.e., the suicide belief sytem) and to rate the relative severity and duration of suicidality and, ultimately, the behavioral response and related change over time. The STR is particularly useful for patients who react primarily to internal triggers, frequently those with recurrent suicide attempts and prominent personality psychopathology. It helps them connect thoughts, feelings, and behaviors in a concrete manner consistent with a CBT conceptualization. In addition, the STR is useful in the treatment process given that, as a result of improving self-monitoring and general emotional awareness, it facilitates a sense of *control* around a topic often identified as *out of control*.

Identifying the content of the SBS is also fairly simple and straightforward. Chapters 5 and 6 go into considerable detail about risk assessment and subsequent monitoring, offering a standard set of questions targeting suicidal

Modal outline: Initial (Date): ____   Revised (Date): ____

Predisposing   *Prior Axis I diagnoses:* _____
vulnerabilities: _____

    Prior Axis II diagnoses: _____
    _____

    Prior suicide attempts (total): _____

    Developmental trauma (summarize):
    _____
    _____

    Family history of suicidal behavior (summarize):
    _____
    _____

    Other factors (summarize): _____
    _____

Identifiable   *Internal (thoughts, images, feelings, physical*
triggers: *sensations):*
    _____

    External (situations, circumstances, places, people):
    _____

    Identifiable themes (e.g., abandonment, rejection):
    _____

Suicidal   **Cognitive triad** (*write out specific beliefs*):
belief   *Self:* _____
system: *Others:* _____
    Future: _____

    Categories (*circle all that apply*):
    Unlovable   Helplessness   Poor distress tolerance

    Conditional rules/assumptions:
    _____
    _____

    Compensatory strategies:
    _____
    _____

(continued)

FIGURE 2.4. Suicidal mode summary worksheet. From *Treating Suicidal Behavior: An Effective, Time-Limited Approach* by M. David Rudd, Thomas Joiner, and M. Hasan Rajab. Copyright 2001 by The Guilford Press. Permission to reproduce this figure is granted to purchasers of this book for personal use only (see copyright page for details).

Affective system

Reported feelings (*circle all that apply*):

Depression   Anxiety   Guilt   Shame

Anger   Sadness   Fearfulness   Embarrassment

Disappointment   Humiliation   Hurt

Other (*list*): _____

_____

Rating of intensity of emotional pain
(1–10): _____

Rating of distress tolerance (1–10): _____

Physiological symptoms:

List arousal symptoms:

_____

_____

_____

Rating of agitation intensity (1–10): _____

Behavioral system:

Current preparatory behaviors
    (*circle all that apply*):

Financial arrangements

Insurance arrangements   Letter writing

Acquiring means to suicide

Detailing a specific plan (how, when, where)

Rehearsal behaviors   Actual attempts

Giving away belongings

Will preparation

Taking steps to guard against rescue

Other (*list*): _____

FIGURE 2.4. *(cont.)*

thinking that can be used in day-to-day practice. For now, we summarize the more general questions that clarify the structural content of the suicidal belief system. What specific type of suicidal thoughts is the patient having? The F-I-D acronym is useful to monitor the characteristic features of any ruminative or obsessive thought process, particularly suicidal ideation. How frequent are the thoughts? How intense? What is the duration of the thoughts? Do the thoughts last a few seconds, minutes, or hours? As discussed in more detail in Chapter 6, it is useful to have the patient rate intensity on a scale of 1 to 10 (e.g., "Would you rate the intensity of your thoughts, that is, how strong or overwhelming they feel, on a scale of 1 to 10, with 1 being not overwhelming at all and 10 being completely overwhelming?"). Ratings are useful for a number of reasons. They provide a sense of control, but, more important, they provide the clinician an accessible subjective measure for comparison and monitoring purposes across sessions (see Chapter 6).

As mentioned previously, the clinician also needs to identify the cognitive triad: the patient's beliefs about self, others, and the future. It is best to keep these questions simple. For example, patients can be asked, How would you describe yourself? How would you describe your family and friends? What kind of a future do you see for yourself? Conditional rules/assumptions and compensatory strategies can be identified by asking the patient *what he or she has done in the past in an effort to feel better*. For example, the patient might manifest avoidance through substance abuse ("I try to numb myself and avoid conflict of any kind by getting drunk"). The clinician can also ask, "What has to happen or what do you have to do in order to feel good?" The patient will likely respond with a common theme such as perfectionism ("If I do everything perfectly, I'll be OK"). Often, this information is offered spontaneously during a standard diagnostic clinical interview and history. Nonetheless, it is important for the clinician to be ready with a standard set of questions to elicit the information necessary to complete the suicidal mode in the event it is not offered spontaneously.

The affective system can be assessed quickly, simply by asking patients how they feel. As becomes apparent in later chapters, it is important to be as detailed as possible, asking patients for a broad range of feelings to capture the essence of the dysphoria to be targeted (see Chapter 6). It is also helpful to gauge severity by asking patients to rate their emotional pain on a scale of 1 to 10 (e.g., "Can you rate the severity of the emotional pain you're feeling now on a scale of 1 to 10, with 1 being minimal and 10 being intolerable?"). Similarly, pain tolerance can also be rated on a scale of 1 to 10 by asking the question "How would you rate your pain tolerance (your ability to tolerate emotional pain) on a scale of 1 to 10, with 1 being very poor and 10 being very good?" As with the other modal components, it is important to explore the presence of patterns or themes across multiple suicide attempts.

An inventory of arousal symptoms is fairly straightforward. In particular, it is important to review those symptoms with empirical support: depression, anxiety, agitation, insomnia, panic, anger, and impaired attention–concentration. As with the other modal components, subjective ratings are also useful for arousal and agitation (e.g., "Could you rate your agitation on a scale of 1 to 10, with 1 being completely calm and 10 being so agitated it is intolerable?"). As noted in Chapter 6, the ratings are not only useful in risk assessment but also allow the clinician to monitor fluctuations in agitation both within and across sessions, providing a more accurate picture of a given patient's emotion regulation and distress tolerance skills. For example, the clinician may quickly discover that despite a patient's being highly agitated early in a session, he or she is calmed considerably, at least to tolerable levels, within only a few minutes and without any complex intervention.

Finally, the behavioral mode is characterized by behaviors in preparation for suicide (planning, rehearsal, financial and insurance arrangements, letter writing) or related self-destructive behaviors and impulsivity (substance abuse, risk taking, sexual acting out). If the patient has a history of multiple suicide attempts, observable patterns will be likely. These patterns can be identified by asking the simple question "What have you done in past suicidal crises?"

A detailed outline of the suicidal mode not only promotes a sense of self-control and lays the foundation for treatment but also allows the practicing clinician to consistently implement a functional analysis of the patient's suicidal behavior(s) across different episodes. This analysis is accomplished by translating the suicidal mode into the patient's *suicidal cycle,* a linear descriptive diagram, each time an attempt or related behavior occurs. Figure 2.5 provides an example of a *suicidal cycle* for a hypothetical patient, Mr. A. The cycle denotes the triggering event, subsequent activation of the suicidal belief system, emotional dysphoria, prominent arousal, and suicidal behavior in order to gain relief. Ideally, the STR can be translated into the suicidal cycle in order to promote self-awareness and identify treatment targets and specific problem areas, as well as to monitor progress over time.

The clinician can simply transfer the patient's descriptions from the STR to the suicidal cycle. As illustrated in Figure 2.5 for Mr. A, his suicidal episode was triggered by his wife's "saying he was worthless." He subsequently "thought she was right" and that "he'd never change," resulting in anger, depression, and guilt. He experienced significant autonomic arousal and "got out his medication, counted them out, and gulped down a beer." Both the STR and the suicidal cycle help the clinician articulate a step-by-step sequence of behavior that can be targeted in treatment, combating the idea that "it happened so fast I didn't know what was going on." As treatment progress is made and the suicidal mode is not as easily activated or is *replaced* by more functional modes, the suicidal cycle changes dramatically. A clear indication of change is the emergence and expansion of nonsuicidal behavioral responses to similar

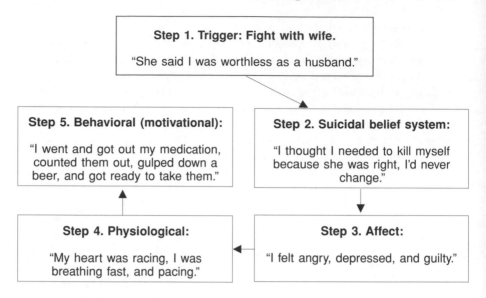

FIGURE 2.5. The suicidal cycle for a single episode: The case of Mr. A.

triggering events, thoughts, and feelings. All these responses are clearly denoted in the suicidal cycle.

Implications of the Suicidal Mode for the Organization, Content, and Process of Treatment

The CBT model offered has some fairly practical implications for the organization, content, and process of treatment. Beck (1996) identified three approaches to treating dysfunctional modes, including deactivating them, modifying their structure and content, and constructing more adaptive modes to neutralize them. This approach, which recognizes the multiple and varied tasks essential to treating suicidality, is consistent with that discussed by Rudd (1998a), which distinguishes between three treatment phases (i.e., crisis, skill building, and personality development), each with a specific treatment agenda and content, despite the existence of considerable overlap. As evidenced by the components of the suicidal mode and the 10 axioms of cognitive theory, cognitive restructuring is only one component of treatment, despite its taking a central role.

The idea is that for the most part, permanent cognitive restructuring cannot occur without activation of the suicidal mode and each component system.

That is, affective experience and mobilization of the mode are essential to treatment progress incorporating meaningful skill development and lasting personality change. Enduring change is structural change, and structural change depends on affective and behavioral impulse, both signifying sincere activation of the mode. In accordance with this model, suicidal crises are a necessary and expected part of treatment, that is, if the suicidal mode is to be permanently altered both in content and threshold for activation as well as in subsequent restriction of the range of potential triggers. Otherwise, initial treatment efforts are likely to focus on facilitating modes that, although critical, are simply not at the core of the suicidal problem. Paradoxically, once suicidality is effectively diffused, the bulk of treatment will address facilitating modes (i.e., enduring personality psychopathology) and the development and refinement of competing and more adaptive modes for living.

Theoretical Flexibility of the Suicidal Mode for Psychotherapy Integration

Aside from the conceptual and clinical advantages summarized previously, the primary strength of the suicidal mode and the CBT model proposed is its flexibility for psychotherapy integration. Alford and Beck (1997) have fully detailed the *integrative power* of cognitive theory and therapy. Their argument holds true for the conceptualization and treatment of suicidality as well. The majority of approaches to the psychotherapeutic treatment of suicidality can easily be integrated into and addressed within the framework offered, including psychodynamic (e.g., Maltsberger, 1986), existential and self-psychology, family systems (e.g., Richman, 1986), and Shneidman's model (1993, 1996) discussing the context of *the suicidal mind.*

For example, Shneidman (1993) distilled existing theory and research down to one simple and definitive statement: "suicide is caused by psychache" (p. 51). More specifically, psychache is defined as "psychological pain in the psyche, the mind" (p. 51). This is an elaboration of his earlier conceptual model of suicide noting the convergence of *pain, perturbation, and press* (Shneidman, 1987). In accordance with this approach, suicide and suicidal behavior are viewed as intrinsically psychological phenomena, a function of individual pain and tolerance; both of which are determined, influenced, and modified by a multitude of factors (e.g., epidemiological, philosophical, sociological, sociocultural, familial, psychiatric, and biological). Shneidman (1996) noted that the practicing clinician can best understand, assess, manage, and treat suicidal behavior by attending specifically to these two variables, the patient's experienced (and expressed) pain and demonstrated pain tolerance. As Shneidman (1987, 1993, 1996) has aptly noted, psychological pain is inextricably tied to psychological/emotional needs (e.g., see Murray, 1938).

Psychache is the result of frustrated psychological needs, and in recognition of the multidimensional nature of suicidal behavior itself, there are innumerable potential causes for the blocked need(s). Shneidman distinguished between modal, or day-to-day, needs and vital needs—those that when frustrated produce intolerable psychological pain and, if unchecked and under the right circumstances, can lead to suicidal behavior or suicide. He also emphasized the variable nature of vital needs from individual to individual but, nonetheless, the consistent fact that we all have psychological/emotional needs that are more important and meaningful than others, and which, when frustrated or blocked, result in more intense psychological/emotional pain.

Shneidman's (1987, 1993, 1996) model can easily be understood within the CBT framework provided. Essentially, he describes the various components of the suicidal mode with a particular focus on affective schemas (i.e., emotional pain and pain tolerance). Suicidal behavior, or behavioral schemas, according to this theory, represent a means of quelling emotional pain and are a function of poor pain tolerance. Other theoretical approaches can similarly be integrated within the CBT model proposed, each emphasizing a different system or component of the suicidal mode.

The Therapeutic Relationship in Cognitive-Behavioral Therapy: Three Fundamental Assumptions

As discussed in Chapter 1, a strong therapeutic relationship and alliance are viewed as essential to therapeutic change in treatment of suicidality. Accordingly, steps need to be taken from the outset to establish an effective relationship and alliance (i.e., agreement between clinician and patient as to the nature of the problem and what to do about it). This is particularly true in time-limited CBT. Although difficult when working with chronically suicidal and personality-disordered patients, it is not an unreasonable or unattainable goal, even in the most brief treatment settings. An active effort needs to be made to maintain this relationship over time, and, accordingly, the relationship needs to be evaluated periodically. It is important to recognize that patients who withdraw prematurely from treatment, or refuse treatment entirely, are often the most severely disturbed (e.g., Rudd, Joiner, & Rajab, 1995).

Responding appropriately requires patience, persistence, and comfort in dealing with hostility and interpersonal aggressiveness. It is important for the clinician to remind him- or herself of a few simple facts about the situation. These *facts* support the fundamental assumptions that guide CBT for suicidality and are consistent with the previous discussion of the *active* suicidal mode and the suicidal belief system.

1. The patient is, more than likely, manifesting serious psychopathology. Translated, this means that as a part of his or her day-to-day functioning he or she is having considerable interpersonal difficulty (i.e., a significant skill deficit). As a result, the patient, more than likely, will have trouble dealing with the clinician too. Not to mention that the clinician is a *safe target* for hostility given the situational dynamics in place. It is a fairly safe bet that the clinician will not respond in hostile or attacking fashion. At a minimum, the expectation the clinician will treat the patient *better than everybody else* is reasonable. As a result, the clinician might well bear the brunt of the patient's anger and hostility.

2. Second, the patient is being seen at his or her worst, that is, when he or she is acutely suicidal. This is a period in which the suicidal mode is active and the suicidal belief system is readily observable. In short, it is important that the treatment mantra be something along the lines of *expect it, prepare for it, and resolve it.* As we will see in Chapter 3, we always have three identifiable agendas operating, including symptom management (crisis resolution), skill building, and personality development. We need to expect these patients to have considerable difficulty; it is simply a function of the problem being targeted.

3. Although the primary emphasis may be on resolving the acute nature of the crisis, it is a wonderful opportunity to initiate skill building and lay the foundation for lasting personality change while simultaneously establishing a solid foundation to therapy. Actually, it can be argued that the hallmark of effective crisis intervention is not only symptom resolution but also skill building and limited personality development. From the very first session, the clinician has an opportunity to establish a model for treatment; that is, he or she will always be addressing multiple targets including symptoms, skills, and personality development. The suicidal mode provides a clear framework for talking about all three. Interpersonal relatedness is a significant part of the problem. Attending to the therapeutic relationship early provides a solid and lasting foundation to treatment. As mentioned earlier, the attachment inherent to therapy with suicidal patients and the hope that surrounds it may well be the only thing that sustains some acutely suicidal patients early in the treatment process.

3

An Overview
of the Treatment Process

When faced with a suicidal patient, the practicing clinician is often left wondering, "What exactly do I do with this patient? How frequently, in what manner, and in what order do I address the myriad presenting problems? What symptoms do I target, and for how long?" Building on the empirical findings reviewed in Chapter 1 and the theoretical foundation provided in Chapter 2, this chapter offers an organizational framework to assist in the weighty task of treating suicidal patients. We have four goals for this chapter. First, we want to provide a clinically accessible summary of treatment tasks (i.e., the *content* of therapy) consistent with existing standards of care and supported by empirical findings. Second, we offer an organizational framework for treatment planning, one that incorporates the various treatment tasks discussed in Chapter 2 and complements the conceptual model offered. Third, we emphasize the varied roles, tasks, demands, and potential limitations of psychotherapy with suicidal patients. And finally, we discuss the complicating role of time and chronicity in treatment planning. Our treatment approach is cognitive-behavioral in the truest sense: cognitive restructuring and skill building go hand in hand. One cannot be done without the other. Skill building is simply a series of behavioral experiments, each providing a critical opportunity for cognitive restructuring and lasting change. Accordingly, the treatment agenda includes a range of cognitive *and* behavioral tasks.

This chapter provides a flexible, comprehensive, and thorough *template* for treatment planning, clinical risk assessment, patient management, and ongoing monitoring. Although the framework offered is most consistent with the theoretical model reviewed in Chapter 2, it is flexible enough to be applied to other theoretical orientations. This is a function of its focus on concrete treatment tasks, as well as the inherent flexibility of cognitive-behavioral theory (e.g., Alford & Beck, 1997). Consistent with the discussion of emerging trends in psychotherapy integration offered by Norcross (1997), the integrative approach described is organized around identifiable problem areas, treatment goals, and related tasks that are uniform across suicidal patients, irrespective of diagnosis (both Axis I and II) and specific symptomatic presentation.

Completing the Clinical Picture: Understanding Severity, Chronicity, and Diagnostic Complexity

Inordinate time constraints in time-limited care demand structure and organization in the treatment process, in planning, in day-to-day application, and in monitoring outcome. In Chapter 2, we discussed six fundamental questions about the patient's suicidality that enable us to articulate the suicidal mode. We wanted to know about the patient's history (i.e., predisposing vulnerabilities), stressors that may have precipitated the suicidal crisis (i.e., triggers), the nature of suicidal thinking (i.e., suicidal belief system), feelings (i.e., affective system), physical symptoms (i.e., physiological system), and suicide-related behaviors (i.e., behavioral system). To complete the treatment planning process, it is critical to think about and be able to answer a few additional probing clinical questions. There are three primary features of the patient's presentation: (1) severity, (2) chronicity, and (3) diagnostic complexity. These characteristic features influence treatment goals, how they are organized and targeted (e.g., what is addressed first, second, third and how much time is devoted to each), and determine the actual duration of treatment itself. The additional questions we need to consider include the following:

- *What is the relative severity of dysfunction or disturbance evidenced by the patient?* In other words, can he or she be managed in outpatient psychotherapy or is a more intensive intervention required first such as hospitalization or day treatment? Is the immediate risk for suicide too high to allow for outpatient treatment? If the patient is at high risk but can be treated on an outpatient basis, do special considerations need to be made such as daily monitoring or a *suicide watch* at home?
- *How chronic is the disturbance? That is, how long has the patient been struggling with suicidality?* How many suicide attempts has he or she made, if any? In other words, we want to make sure we distinguish between ideators, single attempters, and multiple attempters.

- *How complex a behavioral picture is presented?* Is the suicidality compounded by other self-destructive and self-defeating behaviors (e.g., self-mutilation, substance abuse, aggressiveness, and sexual acting out) that will also need to be targeted?
- *How complex is the diagnostic picture presented by the patient in terms of both Axis I and Axis II comorbidity?* In all likelihood, the more complex the behavioral picture, the more complex the diagnostic picture and vice versa.
- *What are the associated domains (i.e., nature) of disturbance?* That is, how is the patient actually impaired? What symptoms, deficient skills, and/or maladaptive personality traits are present?

Depending on the answers to these questions and the patient's suicidal mode, we can start to organize the treatment agenda and determine what goals are important and reasonable within a time-limited framework. From the outset, however, it is critical to recognize that those with severe, complex, and chronic suicidality will most likely require longer-term care. Although the treatment agenda will be the same, it will simply take longer. The duration of care, in most cases, will be complicated by frequent relapses and recurrent crises for those evidencing chronic suicidality. The same organizational framework can be applied but the patient's progression through the various levels of treatment will be slower. As discussed in later chapters, this is a part of the informed consent process that needs to be emphasized when treatment goals are identified, expectations created, and a prospective time line established. This is particularly important for the patient, but it is also an issue for insurance carriers and managed care entities.

Identifying Treatment Components

In accordance with the recent trend in psychotherapy (e.g., Layden, Newman, Freeman, & Morse, 1993; Lerner & Clum, 1990; Linehan, 1993; Linehan et al., 1991; Rudd, Rajab, et al., 1996), suicidality can be viewed as a general construct (see Figure 3.1), with three discernible *domains,* components, or visible manifestations of psychopathology consistent with lower-order factors:

1. Symptoms (i.e., depression, anxiety, hopelessness, suicidal ideation, anger, guilt, panic, etc.).
2. Identifiable skill deficits (i.e., problem solving, emotion regulation, distress tolerance, interpersonal skills, and anger management).
3. Maladaptive personality traits (i.e., consistent with personality disorders as defined by DSM-IV and influencing both self-image and the nature of interpersonal relationships with family and friends).

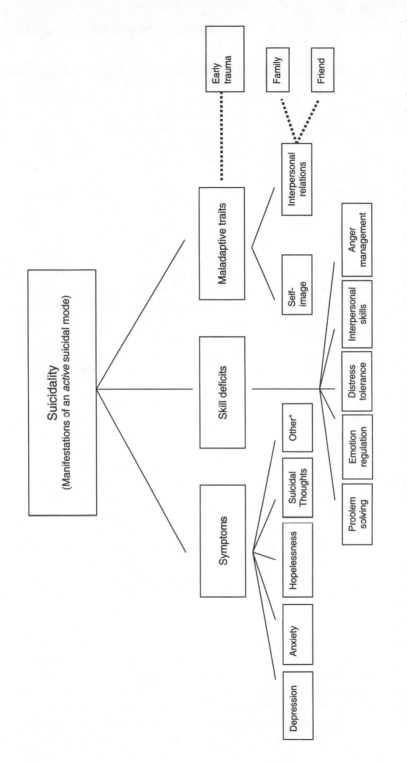

FIGURE 3.1. Conceptualizing dysfunction in suicidality: Higher- and lower-order factors. *Includes guilt, panic, shame, anger, anhedonia, attention/concentration impairment, helplessness, substance abuse, sense of immediacy and urgency, and related behavioral problems such as attempts, self-mutilatory behaviors, high-risk behaviors.

47

Most traditional treatment approaches have focused on symptoms and personality traits, often struggling to integrate the role of deficient skills in a theoretically coherent manner. The most recent approaches have differed, however, emphasizing the three component parts noted previously (e.g., Linehan, 1993; Rudd, Rajab, et al., 1996). These three domains are the essence of what is targeted via psychotherapy, comprising the *content of treatment*. Consistent with the notion of the suicidal mode, each domain is the observable consequence of an *active mode*.

The emergence of managed care entities in the mental health landscape mandate shorter-term, targeted, and symptom-focused treatment. The suicide-specific approaches that have emerged over the last decade are empirically grounded, with identifiable and quantifiable treatment targets. As a result, they are more easily adapted for short-term treatment. Shorter-term and symptom-focused treatment does not, by any means, suggest less effective treatment. As is evident in our previous discussion of the suicidal mode and the interactive and interdependent nature of the modal systems, the more superficial symptoms are related to associated skill deficits and underlying core personality disturbance. All are a part of an active suicidal mode and targeted to some degree during the course of treatment, regardless of duration, and most often in simultaneous fashion. As is apparent from several of the studies reviewed in Chapter 1, brief treatment *can and does* having lasting impact. The end result is, ideally, more efficient and effective treatment and a more precise understanding and measurement of treatment outcome, both in terms of direct and indirect markers of suicidality (see Chapter 4 for a detailed discussion of direct and indirect markers of suicidality). As noted previously, however, those evidencing severe, complex, and chronic suicidality will require longer-term care. One of the benefits of using the treatment-planning framework offered is that it makes it easier to negotiate with insurance companies for additional sessions. Clinicians will be able to discuss in clear and concrete terms what *has and has not* been accomplished in treatment. They will be able to offer a coherent explanation as to why treatment is going to take considerably longer, that is, that the patient's problems are the result of a complex and chronic diagnostic picture compounded by recurrent, severe episodes of suicidality. In essence, the suicidal mode is more active, stable, and easily accessible.

The content of treatment is more readily *accessible* and *quantifiable* as a result of these suicide-specific approaches (as illustrated in Figure 3.1). We can discuss more clearly and cogently what we are actually doing in therapy, what we are working on specifically, and the types of change we expect to occur. We can articulate where we are in the treatment process (i.e., what *component(s)* of treatment we are targeting). We can also monitor and measure this change over time. As discussed later, this conceptualization has led to the identification of treatment tasks that provide a foundation for psychotherapeutic integration and a coherent organizational framework for the treatment of suicidality in a managed care environment.

An Overview of the Goals for Each Treatment Component

As summarized previously, empirically based approaches have incorporated three *treatment components* that target (1) symptoms, (2) deficient skills, and (3) maladaptive personality traits. Couched within the theoretical model of the suicidal mode, these three components form the foundation of our treatment approach (see Figure 3.4 for a summary). In other words, the patient's symptoms, deficient skills, and maladaptive traits are the observable consequences of the active suicidal mode, as well as the facilitating modes during periods in which the suicidal mode is inactive. The general goal is not just to deactivate the suicidal mode but to help the patient develop more adaptive modes, making it much more difficult to activate or trigger the suicidal mode in the future. That is, we want to raise the patient's threshold for becoming suicidal. When the patient is no longer highly symptomatic, is making use of improved skills, is more hopeful about the future, has a restructured suicidal belief system, has an improved self-image, and is functioning better in relationships, a new and more adaptive mode has been developed. Adaptive modes need to be accessible during periods of acute stress and crisis. Although each treatment component cuts across multiple systems of the suicidal mode, each has discrete, identifiable goals along with specific treatment targets. As discussed in more detail later, each treatment component is addressed *simultaneously*, with varying degrees of time and intensity depending on the specifics of the clinical situation.

Goals for Symptom Management

The goals for the symptom management component, focus specifically on acute symptomatology and immediate day-to-day functioning. Among the goals are the following:

- Resolve any immediate crisis.
- Reduce suicidality, including diffusing suicidal thoughts and related behaviors.
- Instill a sense of hopefulness regarding both the immediate future and the treatment process.
- Reduce overall symptomatology.

Goals for Skill Building

Goals for the skill-building component revolve around skill identification, development, and refinement. The task, for the most part, is to identify the patient's current level of functioning, associated skill level, and deficient areas to target and to pursue accordingly. Among the goals are the following:

- Identify current skill level across targeted areas of problem solving, emotion regulation, self-monitoring, distress tolerance (i.e., impulsivity), interpersonal assertiveness, and anger management.
- Improve the patient's general level of functioning, that is, return to premorbid level or better.
- Help the patient develop and refine basic skills in the areas identified as deficient.

Goals for Personality Development

The goals for the personality development component are much broader in focus and, accordingly, are likely to be longer term. Specifically, the goals target three areas: self-image disturbance, developmental trauma, and interpersonal functioning including relationships with family and friends. This component targets more enduring psychopathology, and, naturally, it will be a particularly important aspect of treatment for those evidencing chronic suicidality. Among the goals are the following:

- Improve the patient's overall self-image and sense of esteem (e.g., address persistent sense of self-loathing, guilt, shame, hatred, inadequacy, or incompetence).
- Help the patient resolve internal conflicts, developmental trauma, and underlying *core* issues (e.g., early sexual, emotional, or physical abuse).
- Help the patient improve the quality and nature of his or her interpersonal relationships, including those with both family and friends (e.g., improved intimacy as well as accessibility and quality of support).

An Overview of the Steps in Treatment Planning

As illustrated in Figure 3.2, treatment planning can be summarized in five sequential steps. These steps are straightforward and relatively simple. The first step is to complete the initial interview(s) and related history. As a part of this process, initial risk assessment ratings and diagnoses are determined (see Chapters 4 and 5, this volume, for a detailed discussion of each). The second

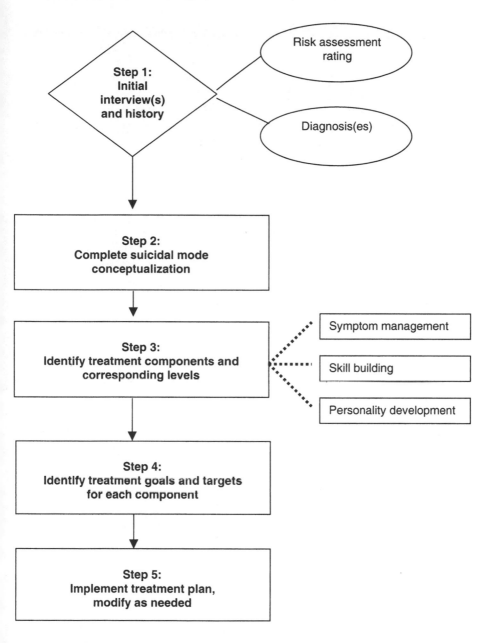

FIGURE 3.2. Treatment planning flowchart.

step is to complete the suicidal mode as reviewed in Chapter 2. This will probably require several interviews. Its completion will assist the clinician in accomplishing step 3: identifying treatment components and assigning corresponding levels, depending on the severity, complexity, and chronicity of the patient's presentation. The next section covers the method for identification and assignment. Once the levels for each treatment component are designated, the corresponding treatment goals and targets in step 4 can be identified using Figure 3.4. Finally, in step 5, the treatment plan is implemented and modified as the patient progresses through the various levels of each treatment component.

The rest of this chapter discusses how to designate levels for each treatment component (step 3), as well as to identify associated goals and corresponding treatment targets (step 4). Later chapters address specific clinical techniques for implementing each component.

Understanding the Treatment Process: Treatment Components and Corresponding Levels

Figure 3.3 summarizes the treatment process. It provides a matrix of treatment components and corresponding levels. As illustrated, the treatment process incorporates three components: (1) symptom management, (2) skill building, and (3) personality development. In addition, each component has corresponding *levels*, indicative of treatment progress within the particular targeted area. The variations in component levels represent therapeutic and individual change and growth over time. Not all suicidal crises are identical. Although Slaikeu (1990) defined crisis as "a temporary state of upset and disorganization, characterized chiefly by an individual's inability to cope with a particular situation using customary methods of problem-solving" (p. 15), the recurrent

Component:

Level	Symptom management	Skill building	Personality development
I	Stabilization	Skill acquisition	Personality stabilization
II	Self-management	Skill refinement	Personality modification
III	Utilization	Skill generalization	Personality refinement

FIGURE 3.3. Matrix of treatment components and corresponding levels.

crises experienced by suicidal patient's vary in nature and quality over time. Nor is skill development or enduring personality change in psychotherapy by any means a uniform process. Patients can and will be at varying levels for each component.

Defining the Component Levels

The levels for each of the components are defined as follows:

Symptom Management Component

Level I—symptom management—is characterized by the need for *external* stabilization, that is, direct intervention on the part of the mental health professional (e.g., phone calls, emergency session(s), and hospitalization). Level II—symptom self-management—is characterized by improved skill level on the part of the patient so that direct intervention is no longer necessary, despite acute emotional upset and dysphoria. Level III—symptom utilization—is characterized by effective management of the crisis on the part of the patient but it is coupled with utilization of the crisis for personal growth and change (e.g., recognition and modification of a specific personality trait or identifiable skill deficit).

Skill Building Component

Level I—skill acquisition—is characterized by early experimentation with a new skill. Level II—skill refinement—is characterized by consistent use of the skill and refinement across specific, targeted circumstances (e.g., assertiveness with a specific person in a specific setting such as one's partner or spouse). Level III—skill generalization—is characterized by consistent use (i.e., planned and unplanned) of a skill and application across a broad range of circumstances (e.g., interpersonal assertiveness at home, work, and related settings).

Personality Development Component

Level I—personality stabilization—is characterized by initial skill acquisition that provides for an improved level of day-to-day functioning, with elimination of extreme suicidal, self-mutilatory, and self-destructive behaviors. Level II—personality modification—is characterized by identification and targeting of specific maladaptive traits (e.g., passive-aggressiveness, dependency, avoidance). Level III—personality refinement—is accomplished in concert with crisis utilization and skill generalization. That is, the patient has experienced some basic changes and is making use of available opportunities to further refine and generalize skills, with enhancement of overall level of day-to-day functioning.

The identification of *components* and *levels* in the treatment process provides necessary structure to the organization of assessment and therapeutic tasks. That is, if the clinician knows a given patient's level for each component, the clinician will know what is being targeted in treatment and what is actually happening from session to session. Take, for example, Level I of the symptom management component. At this level, patients are incapable of self-management. The majority of session time will likely be spent on crisis and symptom management, but treatment will also focus on developing the patient's own basic crisis skills, including self-management. This means that the patient is also working on skill acquisition (skill building component, Level I) and initial personality stabilization (personality development component, Level I). Each component is addressed simultaneously. Given the time constraints of treatment, though, one component will consume more time and energy than the others, depending on the specific clinical context. In the example provided previously, the primary focus would be on crisis stabilization, the secondary focus on skill acquisition, and the tertiary focus on personality stabilization. Take, for example, the following sequence in a series of sessions for a patient with a mild, acute episode of suicidality:

• *Session 1:* The patient presents in acute crisis following a squabble with his wife. He is dysphoric, anxious, and experiencing specific suicidal thoughts. The bulk of the session will address the crisis component of treatment, perhaps the entirety of the session. An effort will be made to reduce the patient's manifest anxiety and diffuse the crisis overlay. To some degree, however, skill building will be emphasized (e.g., improving distress tolerance through activity scheduling such as exercise, relaxation training, or listening to music or problem-solving targeting the marital dispute) along with personality development (i.e., allowing for initial skill acquisition to improve day-to-day functioning).

• *Session 2 (the following week):* The patient is no longer acutely dysphoric. The specific suicidal thoughts have subsided. He is, however, continuing to have nonspecific morbid ruminations, as well as a mixture of depressive and anxiety symptoms. Although symptom management will continue to be important, the focus of the session is likely to shift to skill building and, to a lesser degree, personality development.

Using the matrix of treatment components and levels, the clinician can describe in concrete terms where a patient is in the treatment process, exactly what he or she is working on in terms of corresponding treatment targets (across each component), and what goals lay ahead. This approach is somewhat similar to the use of grade equivalents in identifying reading ability. For example, an eighth-grade level in reading, communicates succinctly whether the child is at the expected level of performance depending on age and education and, if not, the observable deficit. The individual would have a separate grade equivalent for each component of the academic curriculum, be it math, reading, or spelling. Similarly, the patient will have a separate level for each of the three targeted components including symptom management, skill building, and personality development.

In addition, the matrix of treatment components and levels provides a means of communicating this information to other providers and insurance carriers. For example, if we describe a patient as having moved to Level III (utilization) of the symptom management component, Level II of the skill building component, and Level II of the and personality development component, then we know that he or she has:

1. Achieved symptom relief and resolution (e.g., is no longer severely depressed, anxious, angry, hopeless, or actively suicidal). In addition, we communicate that if, in fact, another suicidal crisis does emerge, he or she is capable of effectively managing the crisis without formal intervention of any type.

2. Acquired and can implement a number of new skills (e.g., problem solving, emotion regulation, improved distress tolerance, better interpersonal skills, and more effective anger management) across several targeted circumstances.

3. Modified any number of long-standing maladaptive personality traits (e.g., passive–aggressiveness), improved his or her overall self-image, is more hopeful about the future, and likely resolved some early developmental conflicts that have worked to complicate interpersonal relationships.

4. Made fundamental changes in the identified suicidal belief system (i.e., the notion of cognitive restructuring covered in detail in Chapter 9), a change deemed central to lasting change in the suicidal mode.

Symptom Management Component

Although others have discussed the role of crises in the treatment of suicidal patients (e.g., Layden et al., 1993; Linehan, 1993), they have not offered an organizational framework for conceptualizing and monitoring change in the patient's *crisis experience* over time. Not all crises are the same; their characteristic features and process of resolution can help gauge treatment progress in a more refined manner across episodes. As detailed in both Figures 3.3 and 3.4, the identifiable levels for the symptom management component include: *symptom*

Component:	Symptom management	Skill-building	Personality development
Agenda:	Crisis Intervention and symptom management	Skills	Traits
Goals:	1. Resolve immediate crisis 2. Reduce suicidality 3. Instill hopefulness 4. Symptom reduction	1. Identify current skill level across targeted areas 2. Improve level of functioning, return to premorbid or better 3. Develop or refine basic skills summarized above	1. Improve self-image 2. Resolve internal conflicts, developmental trauma, underlying core issues 3. Improve interpersonal relationships, including family
Therapeutic focus:	Crisis and symptom management	Skill development	Personality development
Levels:	I: Stabilization II: Self-management III: Utilization	I: Skill acquisition II: Skill refinement III: Skill generalization	I: Stabilization II: Modification III: Refinement
Targets:	Symptom relief and crisis resolution:	Skill development:	Self-Image and Interpersonal Functioning: Cognitive Restructuring

	1. Depression
	2. Anxiety
	3. Other identifiable symptoms (i.e., anger, guilt, panic, anhedonia, insomnia, attention-concentration impairment)
	4. Hopelessness
	5. Helplessness
	6. Suicidal ideation
	7. Suicidal behavior
	8. Substance abuse
	9. Sense of immediacy and urgency
	10. Poor distress tolerance, impulsivity
		1. Problem solving:
		  a. Eliminate extreme responding and avoidance
		  b. Develop structured and methodical approach
		  c. Skill acquisition, strengthening, generalization
		2. Emotion regulation
		  a. Learn to identify, understand feelings
		  b. Learn to express constructively
		  c. Learn to moderate feelings
		3. Self-monitoring
		  a. Awareness (labeling of feelings)
		  b. Understanding (normalize experience)
		  c. Responding (more effective regulation)
			1. Hopeless nature of belief system
			2. Identify, explore esteem, and efficacy issues
			  a. Defective, inadequate, incompetent
			  b. Unlovable
			  c. Helpless
			2. Identify, explore developmental trauma
			  a. Abuse
			  b. Neglect
			  c. Abandonment
			3. Identify, explore conflicts within the family and social systems
			  a. Attachment
			  b. Enmeshment
			  c. Detachment, separation

(continued)

FIGURE 3.4. Treatment planning matrix.

Component:	Symptom management	Skill-building	Personality development
Targets: *(cont.)*	Symptom relief and crisis resolution:	Skill development:	Self-Image and Interpersonal Functioning: Cognitive Restructuring
		4. Distress tolerance (i.e., impulsivity) a. Raise threshold for reaction b. Lower reactivity (lessen severity) c. Shorten recovery 5. Interpersonal skills a. Assertiveness: address passivity, avoidance, subjugation b. Attentiveness c. Responsiveness 6. Anger management a. Identify, recognize early signs b. Appropriate, constructive expression c. Empathy, acceptance, forgiveness	
Interventions:	Crisis response plan, treatment log, risk assessment, STR, pharmacotherapy	Individual, group psychotherapy, skills training	Individual, group, and/ or family therapy
Therapist role:	Active/directive	Collaborative	Reflective/supportive
Process task:	Engagement	Attachment	Separation
Process marker:	Past orientation	Present orientation	Future orientation

FIGURE 3.4. *(cont.)*

stabilization, symptom self-management, and *symptom utilization*. A failure to recognize or monitor this qualitative change can result in the loss of subtle but, nonetheless, critical information. Without it, important markers of treatment progress, particularly for those evidencing chronic suicidality, are obscured by the recurrent suicide attempts and related crises common to treatment.

Symptom stabilization is characterized by the need for direct intervention on the part of the mental health professional. As we will discuss in Chapter 7, therapist strategies can include creation of a symptom hierarchy to identify and target the most severe symptoms and creation of a crisis response plan. This plan will involve the introduction of needed skills. *Symptom self-*

management refers to improved skill level on the part of the patient so that direct intervention is no longer necessary. The patient can effectively manage
the crisis on his or her own. The final level, *symptom utilization*, refers not
only to effective management of the crisis but also to use of the crisis as an opportunity for personal growth and change, consistent with, at a minimum, *skill
generalization* and *personality modification* (see discussion of other components later). For example, symptom utilization involves not only effective regulation of emotional upset such as acute anxiety or anger but evidence of skill
generalization from one stressor or circumstance to another (e.g., moving
from resolving recurrent and predictable interpersonal conflicts with a family
member to spontaneous relationship problems at work) consistent with emerging (and it is hoped lasting) personality transformation. Consistent with the
definition offered in the fourth edition of the *Diagnostic and Statistical Manual of Mental Disorders* (DSM-IV; American Psychiatric Association, 1994,
p. 629), a personality disorder is characterized by inflexible, rigid, and problematic traits, which result in social and/or occupational dysfunction. Accordingly, the manifestation of change in the context of crisis is consistent with
identifiable changes in personality structure and organization, despite the fact
that they may well be quite minor in magnitude.

Cycling through Components and Levels

Patients cycle through various levels of a given component multiple times during the course of treatment, in all likelihood, exploring and solving similar
problems in different ways as they build skills and enhance and modify their
self-image and sense of confidence. Actually, for a significant number of suicidal patients it is anticipated that they will experience multiple suicidal crises
during the course of treatment and, accordingly, cycle through various levels
of each component multiple times. Ideally, each successive crisis would be resolved in a more effective and efficient manner.

Figure 3.5 provides an illustration of a hypothetical patient *cycling*
through various levels of the three components over the course of 10 weeks of
treatment. As illustrated, the initial trigger (i.e., the precipitant for his presentation to treatment) is a *fight with his wife* in which she threatens divorce. This
activates the suicidal mode, the patient becomes markedly dysphoric, anxious,
depressed, and actively suicidal (symptom management component, Level I).
His problem is compounded by prominent skill deficits that lead to general
avoidance, a lack of assertiveness, withdrawal, and reliance on alcohol abuse
to regulate his feelings (skill-building component, Level I). The patient sees
himself in a negative light, stating that he is *worthless, incompetent, and incapable of making it* (personality development component, Level I). The initial
therapeutic intervention is intensive but ultimately effective at deactivating the

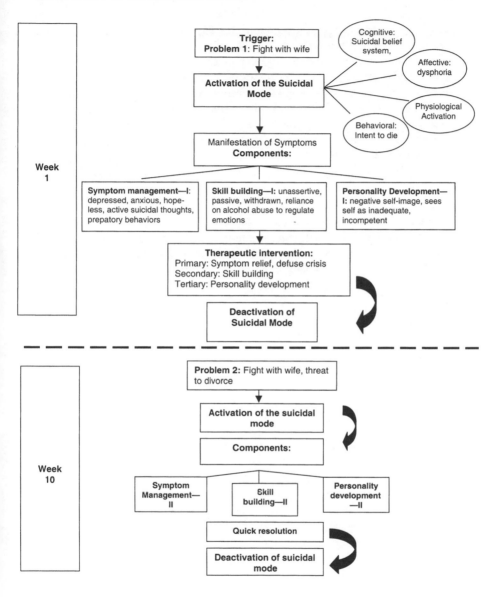

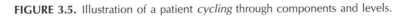

FIGURE 3.5. Illustration of a patient *cycling* through components and levels.

suicidal mode and returning the patient to a baseline level of functioning that enables him to return to work and meet daily demands.

At week 10 during treatment, the patient again has a fight with his wife, activating the suicidal mode. Given progress in therapy, however, the patient is able to manage the crisis himself, experiences only fleeting dysphoria, and much more effectively regulates his feelings without relying on alcohol (symptom management component, Level II). To do so, he implements use of a number of newly acquired skills. He is much more assertive, and instead of withdrawing, he is active and makes a distinct effort to address a number of long-standing marital problems (skill-building component, Level II). The suicidal crisis is relatively brief and not nearly as intense. He and his wife start concurrent marital therapy. As a result of this process, the patient notes a renewed sense of confidence and capability, a feeling that endures well after the crisis has resolved (personality development component, Level II). As this example demonstrates, the same crisis can and, more than likely will, be experienced differently as treatment progresses, skills develop, and personality change evolves.

The Role of Medications

As discussed early in this book, marked comorbidity and diagnostic complexity are, more often than not, the norm in treating suicidal patients. Severe symptomatology is the natural correlate. Remember, we are seeing patients at their worst, in the midst of a suicidal crisis. One of the primary goals of crisis intervention is symptom remission. Frequently, psychotropic medication will be necessary and advised. Aside from issues of diagnosis, the two primary markers that we have used is the degree of impairment in day-to-day functioning and, of course, the patient's wishes. When patients can no longer function and meet the necessary day-to-day demands, medication is often essential to ensure the stability necessary for continuing outpatient care and ongoing psychotherapy. That is one of the benefits of using subjective ratings in assessing risk and symptom severity; they provide an easy marker by which to gauge the patient's level of functioning, change over time, and ultimately progress. Threshold values can be established that, when crossed, signal the need for a medication consultation. These values can be discussed with the patient, and concrete behavioral correlates can be identified and simply monitored over the course of treatment.

From a purely anecdotal perspective, anywhere from 40 to 60% of the patients with whom we work have had, or are currently taking, medication. Frequently, medication is essential to recovery. At other times, this simply is not the case. Accessing medication consultation is a clinical decision best made by the provider and patient on a case-by-case basis. Consistent with this information, we have generally considered the chronicity of the patient's disturbance, the severity of symptoms, and the diagnostic complexity of the presentation. If medication is a component of treatment, it is important to establish and maintain a working relationship with the psychiatrist or physician prescribing. In most cases, periodic and predictable consultation is critical to effective management and treatment.

Skill-Building Component

The levels identified for the *skill-building* component are consistent with conceptualizations offered by others. Among the specific skill areas covered, self-monitoring, distress tolerance, and emotion regulation are believed to be critical for all suicidal patients and represent *core interventions* that will be standard regardless of the particular clinical presentation. Those making multiple suicide attempts and exhibiting chronic suicidal behavior, in particular, have proven distinctive in this respect (e.g., Linehan, 1993; Rudd, Joiner, & Rajab, 1996). They frequently evidence limited emotional awareness (i.e., poor self-monitoring), experience difficulty in recovering when emotionally upset (i.e., emotion regulation), and are often impulsive when dysphoric (i.e., poor distress tolerance). Consistent with one of the central goals of dialectical behavior therapy (Linehan, 1993), considerable effort is expended to raise the patient's threshold for emotional upset, lower his or her reactivity (i.e., intensity of emotional reaction), and shorten the time necessary for recovery. As is evident, there is a clear interrelationship between self-monitoring ability, emotion regulation, and distress tolerance. Essentially, it is posited that the more emotionally aware patients are, the more effectively they will regulate emotion, the greater their tolerance for distress, and the less they manifest impulsivity. Specific skill development in psychotherapy is assumed to progress in a fairly predictable fashion, particularly with suicidal patients, from acquisition to refinement and ultimately generalization across situations and circumstances (e.g., Layden et al., 1993; Linehan, 1993; Nezu et al., 1989). *Skill acquisition* is simply experimentation with a newly identified skill (e.g., assertiveness or problem solving). *Skill refinement* is characterized by consistent use of the skill and refinement across specific, targeted circumstances (e.g., assertiveness with a specific individual such as one's boss in a specific setting such as work). Finally, *skill generalization* is characterized by consistent use of a skill (i.e., planned and unplanned) and application across a broad range of circumstances (e.g., interpersonal assertiveness at home, work, and leisure activities). Skill generalization is confirmation that the skill has been adequately developed, is useful and, most important, accessible when needed.

Of critical importance for skill building is a consistent and methodical approach, regardless of the skill being targeted. A consistent approach will not only help motivate the patient but will also facilitate the process of skill acquisition, refinement, and generalization across various settings. The following steps are suggested:

1. Identify specific skill deficits for the patient and keeping a running log (i.e., self-monitoring either through a journal or daily record of some type).
2. Place the deficit in context, both developmentally and with respect to current functioning (i.e., help the patient recognize and understand the origin of the deficit and implications for day-to-day activities).
3. Identify and explore the potentially recurrent nature of the problem or deficit (i.e., chronicity) over time. Help the patient recognize that the skill deficit probably appears with some regularity. It is particularly important to help patients recognize that the deficit is present much of the time, not just during periods of acute crisis.
4. Identify and address the disadvantages of the deficit(s) (e.g., emotionally, interpersonally, financially, and self-image) to facilitate motivation for change. This can be done easily using a daily journal.
5. Remediate the deficit using a blend of indirect (e.g., education and information) and direct techniques (e.g., role playing and behavioral rehearsal).

Personality Development Component

The personality agenda integrates issues of self-image, interpersonal functioning, and developmental trauma (see Figure 3.4). As detailed in Chapter 2, the principal defining feature of the patient's belief system is hopelessness, a variable which has been consistently linked to suicidality, from ideation to completions (see Weishaar, 1996, for review). Personality trait targets have most consistently revolved around self-image disturbance (i.e., seeing self as defective, inadequate, helpless, and unlovable), developmental trauma and abuse, and interpersonal dysfunction with problems of attachment, enmeshment, and separation, all cloaked within a veil of hopelessness (e.g., Freeman & Reinecke, 1993; Layden et al., 1993; Linehan, 1993). The approaches to addressing personality dysfunction cover a broad range of therapeutic orientations and techniques, with the common feature being the requisite need for long-term contact and a strong therapeutic relationship.

The identified levels for the *personality development* component are also consistent with other conceptualizations of personality change but more specific in nature (e.g., Beck, Freeman, & Associates, 1990). *Personality stabilization* is characterized by *initial* skill acquisition that allows the patient an improved level of day-to-day functioning with elimination of extreme suicidal, self-mutilatory, and self-destructive behaviors, along with noticeable symptom remission. *Personality modification* is characterized by identification and specific targeting of maladaptive traits (e.g., passive–aggressiveness, avoidance, and dependency) while the patient attempts to refine targeted skills and engage in self-management of crises. Finally, *personality refinement* is accomplished in concert with crisis utilization and skill generalization. In other words, the patient has experienced some fundamental and enduring changes, having acquired some targeted skills and applied them with success. He or she is making use of each available opportunity to further refine and generalize skills. The net result is fewer and less severe crises, less intense symptomatology, and improved day-to-day functioning (i.e., both socially and occupationally), ideally, with limited (if any) *active* support on the part of the clinician.

Specific treatment targets from different components are routinely addressed simultaneously, although those from other than the primary component targeted naturally consume less time during sessions (see Figure 3.4). During the symptom management component, for example, not only will acute symptomatology, suicidality, and hopelessness be the focus of intervention, but also their successful resolution will assist in skill building and self-image/personality development.

Variation in Therapist Role

Each component demands variation in the role orientation of the therapist, ranging from directive to collaborative to reflective. The identified treatment components are also hierarchical in nature, that is, in terms of the amount of time devoted to particular agenda items (i.e., targets) during treatment sessions. Specifically, in the symptom management component of treatment, a disproportionate amount of time is spent with crisis intervention tasks, depending on the patient's day-to-day stressors, symptom severity, and individual skill level. Naturally, the role orientation of the clinician is more directive during this beginning component given the crisis intervention nature of treatment.

As the patient establishes an adequate skill repertoire, crises resolve more quickly and effectively, active symptomatology is less of a concern, with a disproportionate shift in time available to address specific skill deficits and target more enduring issues of self-image, interpersonal functioning, and related developmental trauma. Accordingly, a collaborative orientation predominates. As individual skill level develops further, the majority of time in treatment is spent on the longer-term issues noted previously, with limited time devoted to skill refinement and even less time to symptom management and crisis intervention. There is a natural shift in the therapeutic role orientation, taking on more a reflective and supportive position, although active collaboration continues.

A Clinical Example of Acute Suicidality: The Case of Mr. E

The organizational framework offered can be applied easily across the full spectrum of those presenting with suicidality, from the most severe chronic individuals to those presenting with a first attempt. In each case, the primary goal is simply to identify the appropriate components and levels, and focus treatment efforts accordingly.

Background of Case

The patient, a 23-year-old single male, requested evaluation following his arrest for public disturbance and intoxication. Apparently, he was arrested after an argument with his girlfriend in which he "threatened to kill himself." He reported no current suicidal thoughts, stating that they "lasted only a few days" following the breakup of the relationship. The thoughts were described as nonspecific with Mr. E stating, "I never thought how I'd do it." He reported no intent, no actual attempt, and no prepatory behaviors of any type. He also reported no previous suicidal crises and no prior mental health care. The patient described no prominent symptomatology, only brief depression and anxiety "that lasted a few days," consistent with an adjustment disorder with mixed emotional features. He did note episodic alcohol abuse over the last month, stating that he was "drunk" at the time of his arrest but had had nothing to drink since, adding that he "has only been drunk three times in my life." The patient stated that he was in his final year of college, was a "straight A student," and was "planning on getting married" when the relationship abruptly ended. He reported that he "relied heavily" on his girlfriend for support and that "she was the first serious relationship" in which he had been involved. He noted that for the most part, he felt "indecisive" and "had a hard time doing things for himself." He reported occasional problems "controlling anger," stating that he would "yell and make threats." He reported only a few friends and social activities outside of his relationship with his girlfriend but described very "strong attachments" in those few cases.

Initial Treatment Plan

SYMPTOM MANAGEMENT COMPONENT, LEVEL II
(SELF-MANAGEMENT)

The patient is no longer actively suicidal or in acute crisis. He did not make an attempt but noted nonspecific suicidal thoughts and voiced a threat. The symptoms resolved spontaneously without formal mental health intervention. The patient is currently functioning adequately and hopeful about any ongoing treatment. He is currently capable of managing day-to-day activities with no symptomatic problems. This is consistent with his report of no significant problems prior to the current relationship. The majority of the patient's therapy will focus on targeted skill building and personality development as his symptoms have resolved.

SKILL-BUILDING COMPONENT, LEVEL I (ACQUISITION)

The patient possesses limited skills and would require skill training targeting specifically improved self-monitoring (i.e., self-awareness), emotion regulation, distress tolerance, and anger management. Problem solving would be integrated but would likely be secondary to the above given the impulsive nature of his suicidal crisis. The suicidal crises highlighted what, in all likelihood, was a long-standing skill deficit(s). Prior evidence of a problem was probably more subtle and less visible but likely will become more apparent as treatment progresses.

PERSONALITY DEVELOPMENT COMPONENT, LEVEL II (MODIFICATION)

The patient does not present in any acute crisis and notes that this is his first mental health evaluation. Prior to his current presentation, he appears to have adjusted and adapted fairly well (e.g., college grades, no previous problems). However, he does evidence some maladaptive personality traits that would be the focus of ongoing work. Personality components that would naturally be woven into ongoing interventions would include (1) poor self-image, (2) lack of confidence, and (3) marked in dependency in relationships.

Mr. E presents a symptomatic picture evidencing spontaneous resolution and requiring no acute intervention and no specific symptom management. Essentially, his suicidal crisis appeared to be the function of limited skills (i.e., self-monitoring, emotion regulation, distress tolerance, and anger management) and related personality dysfunction (i.e., prominent dependency). In his case it may well be that targeted intervention can result in lasting change.

The case of Mr. E. can be summarized with relative ease using the treatment planning matrix. Each treatment component can be understood in terms of specific treatment goals and targets. The treatment planning matrix is an excellent tool for summarizing the treatment process and treatment components; identify corresponding goals and targets; translating the treatment agenda to the patient, fellow clinicians, and insurance administrators; and monitoring treatment progress and the process of individual change.

Monitoring the Treatment Process

Essentially, the treatment process (i.e., movement through the levels of each treatment component) can be accurately gauged and monitored by the content (i.e., treatment agenda and associated assessment and treatment targets or tasks) of therapy, not its duration. The important point with respect to this conceptual and organizational framework is that an individual successfully treated for suicidal behavior will transition through the same component levels (treatment process), regardless of the duration of treatment. He or she will address the same treatment agenda(s) and specific target areas, simply in a different time frame and potentially by a different mechanism of action (i.e., the specific psychotherapeutic model employed). Where the patient is in the treatment process can be addressed rather simply: What do you spend the majority of your session time discussing and targeting?

The organizational framework offered provides a means of more clearly articulating where a patient is in the treatment process. Each patient can be placed within the treatment process by describing both components and corresponding levels. This translates into a clearly articulated treatment agenda with respect to active symptomatology being targeted, particular skills being developed, and enduring personality traits being explored.

Figure 3.6 provides a worksheet for monitoring treatment components and levels. It is recommended that the worksheet be completed at various points during the treatment process, specifically at intake, during periodic planned reviews (e.g., when a treatment *update* is requested by an insurance carrier), when referred to another provider, and at treatment completion or termination. It is particularly important if termination is unplanned. For example, if a patient abruptly discontinues treatment (i.e., voluntary withdrawal), it is critical to log the patient's progress to date and level of functioning when he or she withdrew from treatment. Completion of the component and level worksheet provides a clear and concise summary of the patient's level of functioning at any one point in time. All the clinician needs to do is to circle the levels for each treatment component. There is also room for relevant clinical notes. As illustrated, it provides a fairly concise means of addressing current level of functioning, severity of psychopathology, and related treatment goals in comprehensive fashion.

Process Tasks and Markers

As detailed in Figures 3.4 and Figure 3.7, the clinician and patient move through a process of engagement, attachment, and separation not only in each individual session but also throughout ongoing treatment. The clinician can

Treatment point (circle one):	Intake assessment
	Periodic review, No. of sessions _____
	Transition or referral
	Termination, planned
	Termination, unplanned (e.g., abrupt discontinuation)

Symptom management component (circle one):	Level I: Symptom stabilization
	Level II: Symptom self-management
	Level III: Symptom utilization
Current target(s):	

Skill building component (circle one):	Level I: Skill acquisition
	Lovol II: Skill rofinomont
	Level III: Skill generalization
Current target(s):	

Personality development (circle one):	Level I: Personality stabilization
	Level II: Personality modification
	Level III: Personality refinement
Current target(s):	

Notes:

FIGURE 3.6. Treatment component and level worksheet. From *Treating Suicidal Behavior: An Effective, Time-Limited Approach* by M. David Rudd, Thomas Joiner, and M. Hasan Rajab. Copyright 2001 by The Guilford Press. Permission to reproduce this figure is granted to purchasers of this book for personal use only (see copyright page for details).

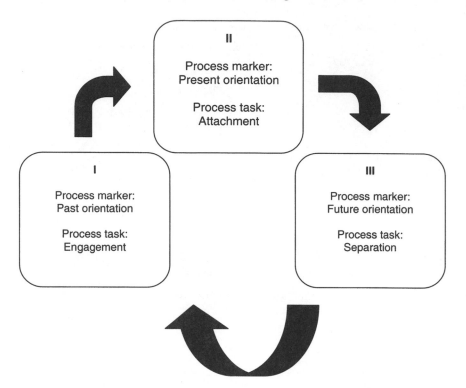

FIGURE 3.7. The treatment process: Stages and characteristics.

monitor this process by attending to *content markers* during and across sessions. Specifically, in the symptom management component of treatment, the majority of the content of a session or sessions will be past oriented as the patient addresses recent or remote emotionally painful issues (the majority of session time spent addressing the ending of relationship, job loss, financial problems, etc.). In the skill building component of treatment, the focus shifts to current functioning, with an emphasis on identifiable skill deficits. Although historical and developmental issues are addressed, the majority of time is likely to be spent on current skill building. Similarly, in the personality development component of treatment the focus shifts to future goals, integrating developmental trauma and previous interpersonal conflicts. Although ideally the patient will have improved his or her level of awareness and understanding for developmental issues that are relevant and targeted identifiable skill deficits, the focus of treatment is likely to revolve around improving self-image and interpersonal functioning through *future* activities, not a perpetual rehashing of old problems.

As is the case across the course of treatment, each individual session mimics the process of engagement, attachment, and separation. Again, the actual content of therapy allows for monitoring of process. For example, early in session, the patient will discuss past issues (e.g., past week functioning and homework assignment(s)), will eventually transition to current functioning and related agenda items, and ultimately will establish an agenda for the coming days, weeks, or month(s). Essentially, each session models the skill of appropriate attachment–separation (i.e., independent functioning) in relationships. This is one of the primary benefits of applying the proposed organizational framework, an improved ability to identify and monitor what are, often, subtle skills and process markers that can be lost in the psychotherapeutic milieu. Such skills are, nonetheless, *critical* to treatment success and important indirect markers of treatment outcome. A clinical example illustrates this process.

The Case of Ms. D, to be discussed in detail later, provides a good example of process variables in treatment. Upon initial presentation, Ms. D discussed in great detail *past* relationships and *past* failures.

THERAPIST: Please tell me about your *current* relationship(s).

MS. D: I'll never have a good relationship with a man, none of them have ever worked out. They've all been failures [past orientation]. The first one ended after only a year, the second one lasted five years, and look what happened to this last one! I've always been a loser in relationships and always will be. I couldn't make one work if my life depended on it.

After facilitating the process of initial *engagement*, however, Ms. D was more open and amenable to discussing her *current* level of functioning, with an identifiable move into the *attachment* phase (i.e., for this initial session). She described current symptomatology in great detail, including suicidal thoughts and behaviors and depressive symptoms, as well as her current drinking pattern. After a thorough evaluation and assessment, the session ended with Ms. D discussing her plans for the immediate future and active participation in treatment, consistent with the *separation* phase (and future orientation).

THERAPIST: Let's discuss and review your plans for the next several weeks.

MS. D: Well, I've got an appointment with you next week and I'll see the psychiatrist tomorrow about medication. Then, I guess, I'll be coming in every week for the next couple of months [future orientation]. Didn't we agree to work on my ability to tolerate feeling bad first, like when I cut myself. I'm feeling OK about doing this, maybe it'll work [hopefulness consistent with future orientation].

Provocations and Resistance
in the Therapeutic Relationship:
How a Clear Organizational Framework Helps

The conceptual and organizational framework offered allows the therapist to specifically target relationship skills that are manifest in the therapy process. As Rudd et al. (1995) and Rudd and Joiner (1998a) have discussed, help negation (including provocations and resistance) in treatment for suicidality is a serious concern, one that requires a compassionate and sensitive approach to transference–countertransference problems. Framing these somewhat abstract concepts as relationship *skills* has numerous advantages in treatment, allowing them to be discussed with the patient in a meaningful and understandable way from the outset.

1. It externalizes the problem to some degree, labeling it as a skill rather than an individual defect of some type.
2. It makes it conceptually easier to grasp and discuss, translating it into a concrete task.
3. It provides a means for monitoring and gauging progress over time. Chapter 9 provides a detailed discussion of the therapeutic relationship.

Quantifying Change: How to Measure and Monitor
Change in Treatment

Measuring change in the treatment of suicidal behavior depends on a range of factors. First, it is essential to use a standard nomenclature for distinguishing what is suicidal and what is self-multilatory and self-destructive. Without such a nomenclature, treatment progress is almost impossible to gauge and monitor. Second, it is important to distinguish between direct and indirect markers of suicidality. Third, it is essential to distinguish between acute and chronic variables in the suicidal process. If these factors are addressed, a general and useful framework can be established and maintained to monitor the progress of the suicidal patient.

In terms of nomenclature, we recommend that the one proposed by O'Carroll et al. (1996) and reviewed in Chapter 1 be universally adopted. Without question, it represents the best the field of clinical suicidology has to offer. It clearly differentiates between suicide attempts and instrumental suicidal behavior, something critical to accurate risk assessment and effective treatment. The notion of direct and indirect markers of suicidality in treatment outcome is a concept that, surprisingly, has not been previously addressed. It is critical to distinguish between the two, particularly given that as direct markers of suicidality improve acute risk wanes, whereas indirect markers might well endure for years.

Direct markers are fairly straightforward and include suicidal ideation (frequency, intensity, duration, and specificity) and suicidal behaviors (attempts and instrumental behaviors). Indirect markers range from symptomatic variables (e.g., hopelessness, depression, anxiety, impulsivity, and anger) to individual characteristics (e.g., attributional style, cognitive rigidity, and problem-solving ability) to personality traits (i.e., in accordance with DSM-IV). Direct and indirect markers of suicidality can be monitored and assessed in a number of ways. Of importance, however, is the need to balance and integrate subjective and objective measures using available psychometric instruments during the course of treatment. Distinguishing between direct and indirect makers of suicidality allows the clinician to differentiate between acute and chronic variables in the suicidal process. Consistent with the conceptual and organizational framework offered, clearly articulating chronic variables helps establish reasonable expectations regarding the treatment process and outcome, facilitates more accurate risk assessment, and lends itself to a reasonable standard of care.

Treatment Withdrawal and Noncompliance

Treatment withdrawal is a fairly common problem with this population, with withdrawal rates of 30% or more across most studies (e.g., Rudd, Joiner, & Rajab, 1995). This is not particularly surprising given that suicidality is, at one level, about ambivalence. The ambivalence about whether to live or die naturally plays out in the course of therapy. In our study, we found that those who withdrew likely did so not because they had recovered and experienced symptom remission but because of prominent personality disturbance that made the intimacy of the therapeutic relationship untenable for many reasons.

Treatment withdrawal can be minimized if adequate informed consent procedures are followed from the very beginning. Being specific and detailed not only will help patients answer questions about issues of *commitment to treatment* but also will help them resolve ambivalence about living. The procedures covered in Chapter 7 provide a framework to ensure that the patient has an adequate understanding and reasonable expectations about the treatment process. If compliance becomes an issue, it needs to be made the primary agenda item until effectively resolved. Otherwise, it can derail treatment, potentially creating a conflictual environment that may only serve to exacerbate the patient's suicidality. Chapter 9 provides a detailed discussion of addressing resistance and noncompliance, couching it within the rubric of the therapeutic relationship.

When patients abruptly terminate or withdraw from treatment, follow-up of some sort is strongly encouraged. We have had considerable success with patients returning to treatment (or at least continuing treatment elsewhere) by simply contacting the patient either by phone or letter (sometimes both) to discuss the reasons for termination and what he or she plans on doing in the immediate future. Sometimes the patient will cite financial problems or time constraints, but, more likely, abrupt withdrawals are secondary to a problem in the therapeutic relationship. We recommend a telephone call for patients who have been in treatment for more that one or two sessions. If the clinician is unable to contact the patient, a simple follow-up letter is best (see Figure 3.8).

Regardless of the circumstances, it is important to *close* a patient's clinical chart with some indication that the closure has been discussed with the patient or an effort has been made to contact him or her to do so. If a patient is unwilling to continue in treatment, it is important to provide other alternatives (i.e., referral to other resources in the local community). The clinician should always document the circumstances surrounding withdrawal, termination, or referral to another provider. In addition, when abrupt termination has occurred, the clinician should always document efforts to contact the patient (either by phone or letter) to coordinate ongoing care. If a letter was sent, the clinician should include a copy in the chart.

Ensuring Treatment Fidelity

Although treatment fidelity is always a concern, the hallmark of this book is its flexibility. It is designed for the practitioner, regardless of setting. The procedures discussed and the framework provided can be implemented anywhere, whether a clinician is operating solo or in a large clinic or hospital. Treatment fidelity is less of an issue for the solo practitioner. For those working in settings with a greater number of clinicians and more resources, treatment fidel-

---

Dear _____:

It has been a few weeks since your last appointment. Given that I haven't heard from you (or have been unsuccessful in reaching you by phone), I simply wanted to touch base to see if all was well. If you'd like, you can give me a call at XXX-XXXX to discuss your plans for future treatment. If you have any questions, concerns, or simply need a referral of any type please let me know and we'll get it arranged. Again, I hope all is going well and I look forward to hearing from you.

Sincerely,

FIGURE 3.8. Follow-up letter.

ity becomes a concern, particularly if a group(s) component is integrated. In these cases, the easiest way to ensure treatment fidelity is by incorporating treatment team meetings with a regular review of procedures, training sessions, and periodic review and discussion of videotaped sessions.

Termination: When, Why, and How

Ideally, termination occurs when patient and therapist agree that the treatment goals have been accomplished. As is evident, treatment of suicidal patients, and particularly chronically suicidal patients, is neither that clear nor that simple. Others have written in some detail about the role of provocation and acting out in the treatment process (see Newman, 1997, for review). In addition, the importance of ensuring that a patient's ongoing treatment needs have been addressed has been stressed by clinicians and researchers alike (e.g., Simon, 1987; Stromberg et al., 1988). The treatment of suicidal patients has been characterized by relatively high withdrawal rates, with those abruptly stopping treatment often continuing to experience marked symptomatology and continued high risk (Rudd et al., 1995).

The organizational framework allows for relatively straightforward assessment of the treatment process, along with markers of acute and chronic risk. Accordingly, it provides some structure and guidance to potential termination issues. Barnett (1998) has offered a number of recommendations regarding appropriate termination. Among them is the need to be specific and clear about expectations from the outset, something facilitated by the framework summarized in Figure 3.4. Moreover, it provides a means of identifying and clearly articulating the need for continued treatment, and in what specific areas. Finally, use of the organizational framework provided allows for clear documentation of the overall clinical picture, treatment goals and targets, accompanying rationale, and monitoring change and progress. As Barnett (1998) noted about termination, "plan for it, prepare for it, and process it" (p. 22). We would add one additional caveat: Simply organize the entire process in a manner meaningful and understandable to patients.

Interpersonal Process Groups and Booster Sessions

As we discuss in Chapter 10, psychoeducational groups can be helpful in skill building. Traditional process groups can also play an important adjunctive role in the treatment process. They can provide the patient an interpersonal outlet to complement ongoing individual therapy. However, it is important that these groups use the same theoretical framework (i.e., the suicidal mode) to complement rather than conflict with ongoing individual work. We have most frequently used the process-oriented groups as an open-ended group to which the patient has access *after* individual treatment is completed. Some clinicians believe that the group is most appropriate only after completing individual treatment; we tend to fall into this category given our reliance on concurrent psychoeducational and problem-solving groups (see Chapter 10). It is recommended that the patient *not* participate in any more than one group activity while simultaneously involved in individual treatment. It can simply be overwhelming to the patient in many ways—emotional, financial, and practical. In the past, we have had patients involved in the psychoeducational group first, followed by the problem-solving group. We have found the process group most helpful as a supportive resource *after* individual treatment is completed. If the process group is accessed after treatment has been completed, it essentially serves the role of *booster sessions*, helping the patient to sharpen skills, provide support, or simply target a specific problem before it escalates.

The Role of the Treatment Team

This book is designed to be flexible. The treatment model can be implemented in a broad range of settings from the sole practitioner to the large group practice. In many settings, such as those with limited resources, the development and use of a treatment team will not be possible. However, if the necessary support is in place, it can facilitate treatment provided by multiple providers within the same institution. The integration of a group component or complement in a particular setting will be enhanced by the development of a treatment team. The treatment team consists of all clinicians treating suicidality in a setting who refer to the group(s). As noted previously, it is recommended that the patient *not* participate in more than one group activity at a time. For those patients involved in individual treatment, it is most effective is to have the patient first complete a psychoeducational group in order to establish basic knowledge and understanding, followed by the problem-solving group, and finally the process group as an ongoing supportive resource. A rotational schedule needs to be established for coherency and coordination in the treatment process.

  If the groups are rotational (e.g., on a quarterly schedule), the group leader can rotate among staff. We have found it most effective and appropriate to have the group leader serve as the team leader, a position that rotates as the groups rotates (e.g., quarterly). If a process group is used in any capacity, it is necessary to have the facilitator's tenure considerably longer (e.g., a year) in duration. If an ongoing process group is in place, the facilitator should not be the team leader given that most patients will likely have completed individual treatment. Moreover, the process group facilitator will have a longer tenure than do the facilitators of the quarterly psychoeducational or problem-solving groups. The team can meet monthly with a specific goal of reviewing all patients' progress, addressing both group and individual issues. The treatment team serves many functions including the following:

- Informing individual clinicians of patients participation in group and issues that are relevant to individual therapy.
- Providing a mechanism for discussion and consultation about difficult cases, particularly those not evidencing progress.
- Support for clinical staff.
- Education and training for staff.
- Staff supervision needs, if appropriate.

In short, use of a treatment team is highly recommended. Actually, without it, treatment of more than one or two highly suicidal patients can be risky and a potentially serious emotional drain on the clinician.

The Need for Long-Term Care in a Time-Limited World

Treating suicidality often times requires considerable time and energy, frequently more time than provided by the insurance carrier. The framework provided here is specific and detailed. Accordingly, we hope it will make it easier for the clinician to make the argument for more enduring care. We have found that if a specific, logical, and detailed argument addressing the patient's risk factors and treatment needs is provided in an understandable format, it is well received. Although the duration of treatment is, without question, more limited now than ever before, we believe we have provided an approach that will make arguments for longer-term care much more effective.

II

ASSESSMENT AND TREATMENT

4

Treatment Course and
Session-by-Session Guidelines

Our treatment model allows the clinician considerable latitude in terms of the overall structure and sequence of therapy. In this chapter, we recommend a general structure and sequence based on the scientific research and theoretical model of suicidality presented earlier, as well as on our clinical experience garnered over the years. The session-by-session guidelines offered here will help practitioners *put it all together* in a coherent but flexible sequence for time-limited treatment. Effective treatment of suicidality demands a broad range of therapeutic skills and techniques. In Part II of this book, we discuss the specific skills and related techniques mentioned here in more depth and emphasize the variable nature with which they are likely to be applied in psychotherapy. This chapter introduces a number of strategies for the first time. Among them are the following: treatment log, symptom matching hierarchy, crisis response plan, ICARE (Identify, Connect, Assess, Restructure, Execute) model of cognitive restructuring, hierarchy of core beliefs, philosophy-of-living statement, and skills deficiency hierarchy. They are all described in much more detail in the following chapters.

It is important to recall that in accordance with our model, the following seven assumptions form the foundation of the treatment process:

1. Suicidality (or an *active* suicidal mode) can be thought of as having three lower-order factors (the identified treatment components) including symptoms, skills deficits, and maladaptive personality traits.

2. Effective treatment includes not only *deactivating* the suicidal mode but also establishing more *adaptive modes,* consistent with the idea of skill building.

3. Imminent risk of suicide is an acute clinical phenomenon, even for those evidencing chronic suicidal behavior. Therefore, imminent risk will endure for relatively brief periods (e.g., hours, days, or a week). The bulk of psychotherapeutic treatment, then, revolves around addressing the underlying *causes* of suicidality, including the *suicidal belief system*, related skill deficits, and maladaptive personality traits.

4. Each treatment component is addressed, at least to some degree, in each and every session, but is done so in hierarchical fashion. That is, more time will be devoted to some treatment targets relative to others depending on the specifics of the clinical presentation and the duration of care.

5. Each treatment component will show identifiable markers of progress consistent with the concept of *levels* for symptom management, skill building, and personality development.

6. Cognitive restructuring is central to treatment success and should be started in the first session and continued throughout the entirety of treatment, regardless of the specific target. Whether targeting symptoms, skills, or maladaptive traits, there are *beliefs* that correspond to each.

7. Time-limited treatment will most often eliminate acute symptoms and result in cognitive restructuring and important changes in the suicidal belief system as well as some initial skill building, but longer-term care will likely be required for enduring personality change.

Couched within these fundamental assumptions, this chapter provides session-by-session *guidelines* and a few clinical examples as illustrations. For the most part, this chapter attempts to describe a *typical* but complex case. It is important to remember, though, that the idea here is to offer a treatment approach that is flexible and applicable across a broad range of clinical settings and circumstances. One of the paradoxical features of suicidality is that there is considerable variability in the contextual factors of the presentation. People become suicidal for many reasons. There are identifiable consistencies, however, across each and every presentation. It is those very consistencies that comprise the *suicidal mode* and make a structured but flexible approach possible.

Consistent with the time-limited theme of this book, the session-by-session guidelines cover a total of 20 sessions that could conceivably be completed over a period of approximately 6 months. This is not an unreasonable amount of time for an individual to be in treatment for suicidality, be it acute or chronic in nature. General guidelines are offered for each session, along with a discussion of how they would apply to a particular case, that of Ms. D. Partial transcripts of sessions are integrated when possible in an effort to clarify how specific goals can be accomplished, topics presented, and issues addressed.

The Beginning of Treatment: Sessions 1–4

As with any psychotherapy, the beginning of treatment is critically important. This is particularly true in a CBT approach. The first few sessions establish the general framework for treatment, help set therapeutic expectations, and provide an opportunity to forge a solid therapeutic alliance. We recommend use of an *extended evaluation period.* As discussed in Chapter 5 (this volume) the period of initial interviews may well take up to four sessions. The purpose of the initial interviews is really quite simple. It provides both the clinician and patient time to complete the initial assessment process in order to accurately understand risk, develop a thorough understanding of the patient's history including diagnosis and prior treatment, complete any initial psychodiagnostics, offer a conceptual model for therapy, and gain informed consent. Essentially, this extended evaluation period provides both the clinician and patient an opportunity to come to an agreement as to whether this particular treatment approach is best and whether the patient can make a commitment to the treatment process. It is difficult, if not impossible, for the patient to make a realistic commitment to treatment without a thorough understanding of just what treatment will involve and what is expected. This is particularly important for individuals presenting with chronic suicidal behavior. Those with chronic suicidality will often have very complex histories, not only in terms of the diagnostic picture presented and problems of comorbidity but also with respect to prior treatment successes and failures.

As discussed in detail in Chapter 5 (this volume), the goals of the initial interviews and this extended evaluation period can be grouped into four categories: risk assessment, treatment conceptualization and consent, consultation and psychological testing, and the therapeutic relationship. Identifiable goals within each category need to be achieved before moving forward with treatment. Risk assessment is an important and continuing task throughout treatment. Accordingly, a risk severity rating needs to be documented for each and every session (see Chapter 5; this volume). Accomplishing these goals within a four-session structure can be challenging, but we have found it a reasonable framework and have not experienced particular difficulty in making it work.

Session 1 Agenda

Two things need to be accomplished during Session 1. First, the clinician needs to assess risk and diagnose. Second, the clinician needs to intervene to diffuse the suicidal crisis and related symptoms. As evidenced later, the nature of the interventions are often fairly simple for the first session. Some strategic interventions are amazingly effective at diffusing acute emotional upset and feelings of *being out of control*. They may involve some basic problem solving: providing the necessary referrals for medication/psychiatric evaluation, implementing patient use of a treatment log and self-monitoring, and scheduling a designated number of appointments.

ASSESSMENT AND DIAGNOSIS GOALS

- Review the patient's history, symptom picture, current suicidal crisis, and develop an initial diagnostic impression (both Axis I and II).
- Complete the initial risk assessment and identify the risk category and initial severity rating as detailed in Chapter 5 (this volume).
- Interview available family members, if at all possible and agreeable to the patient, to assist in the risk assessment process and possibly ongoing management if risk is deemed high.

INTERVENTION GOALS

- Target symptom management and diffuse the current suicidal crisis. This will likely involve some limited problem solving (see Chapter 10, this volume), the possible use of a *symptom matching hierarchy* and formulation of a crisis response plan discussed in Chapter 7 (this volume).
- Initiate use of a treatment log (i.e., to facilitate cognitive restructuring). It is recommended that the patient create a treatment log from the very first session. This log can take many forms, but the most simple is to have patients create (or have the clinician provide) a bound notebook of some type. The notebook should be used in every session. All homework assignments, coping cards, and handouts should be kept as part of the notebook as well. Patients should be encouraged to make an entry at the end of each session, drawing pertinent conclusions about the session. Most frequently, these conclusions will revolve around aspects of the patient's suicidal belief system and related self-image issues. The patient should be encouraged to make use of the treatment log throughout the course of treatment, accessing it during crises as well as simply reviewing it from time to time. We also encourage patients to journal in their treatment log, complete STRs, and keep a list of questions they have and need to address in session. In short, the treatment log should be a repository for all issues addressed in treatment. It provides a lasting and accessible resource for the patient outside therapy and away from the therapist. The treatment log should include a number of component parts. It should help the patient articulate and document any conclusions at the end of the first session. In particular, it is im-

portant for patients to target beliefs not only about self, others, and the future (the suicidal belief system) but also about distress tolerance and the broader concept of emotion regulation. It is important to remember that for skills targeted, patients should be able to articulate a specific belief. All these beliefs are vital to understanding and restructuring the patient's suicidal belief system.

- Negotiate with the patient for an extended evaluation period, at the end of which the patient and clinician will make a definitive decision about the nature of ongoing treatment.
- Schedule the next three sessions.
- Provide a referral for a psychiatric and/or medication consultation if indicated.
- Devise and document a crisis response plan as discussed in Chapter 7.

THE CASE OF MS. D

The patient, a middle-aged, recently separated and twice divorced white female, presented for evaluation reporting that she had been acutely suicidal over the course of the last 2 weeks but had struggled with suicidality much of her adult life. She noted specific suicidal thoughts about shooting herself. She reported having thoughts about 10 times a day but described them as enduring "only for a few seconds" and that she "didn't intend on doing anything about them." The patient reported no prepatory behaviors of any type and noted that she did not own or have access to a gun. She did, however, report three previous overdose attempts, all with no follow-up medical care or psychiatric hospitalizations. She also noted a 20-year history of chronic suicidality with recurrent self-mutilatory behavior, reporting that she would cut on her arms and legs (i.e., in areas covered by clothing so that others would not notice) with a razor blade to "relieve tension." The patient reported that she had been experiencing extensive depressive symptomatology for 2 months since the breakup of her marital relationship. Specifically, she reported persistent depressed mood, anhedonia, weight loss of 20 pounds, insomnia, some agitation, poor energy and fatigue, feelings of worthlessness, and diminished attention–concentration. She also noted episodic alcohol abuse, which has been chronic in nature, but most recently was taking the form of binge drinking over the weekends. She reported feeling "guilty and ashamed" about childhood sexual abuse and "worthless most of the time." In particular, she noted feeling hopeless and angry about her marriage, stating, "This is my third failed relationship, I don't think I'll every have a decent marriage." She reported that she felt "angry all the time" about her estranged husband and was having trouble "controlling it," often "blowing up at people at work." She reported few friends and social activities outside her work environment.

For Ms. D, Session 1 was relatively straightforward. After reviewing her history and current symptomatic presentation, the clinician arrived at a tentative diagnostic impression with considerable comorbidity: Axis I: major depressive disorder, recurrent; posttraumatic stress disorder, chronic; alcohol abuse, episodic; and Axis II: borderline personality disorder. Ms. D's risk assessment category was designated as *chronic high risk with acute exacerbation* and her risk severity rating was 4 (severe). The primary reason her rating was not extreme was because of the absence of active intent in terms of either subjective report or current objective markers of suicidality. As noted, Ms. D was having frequent and specific suicidal thoughts, but they were relatively fleeting in nature and there was no stated intent. Family members were not available and could not be integrated into risk monitoring efforts. Accordingly, Ms. D agreed to *telephone monitoring* over the course of the week. She agreed to check in by phone each day at a designated time to assess her risk and the need for intervention or changes in the treatment plan. We use telephone monitoring quite a bit. It is a straightforward means of monitoring risk in outpatient settings. It is not particularly time-consuming, it is easy to implement and effective, and patients are quite agreeable to using it as an alternative to more intensive interventions such as day treatment or brief hospitalization.

In terms of intervention, a symptom matching hierarchy was completed to identify the most problematic symptoms for intervention, Ms. D noted that among her current symptoms the insomnia and poor appetite were the most disruptive. She agreed to a sleep hygiene protocol which included abstaining from any alcohol use, establishing a standard sleep–wake cycle, eliminating caffeine after her evening meal, and a structured set of activities prior to bed each evening (e.g., reading for 30 minutes and listening to a relaxation tape). In addition, Ms. D was scheduled for a medication consultation and a daily activity schedule was implemented which integrated brief, but daily, exercise (see Chapter 10, this volume).

A crisis response plan was written out on the back of a business card and Ms. D carried the card with her and agreed to make use of it over the course of the coming week (see Chapter 7, this volume). Given that Ms. D was still somewhat dysphoric during the session, the card was actually written for her (although she was active in discussing the steps that could be taken to diffuse a crisis). Sometimes this is necessary. It is not uncommon that a patient in acute crisis will not actively want to write things down in the middle of a session. However, we have consistently been impressed by the number of patients who respond in a positive fashion to opportunities to take active and self-directed roles in their treatment.

The concept of an extended evaluation period was presented to Ms. D, along with the use of a treatment log. The idea of an extended evaluation period can be presented in a nonthreatening fashion and we have actually found that it tends to facilitate motivation and commitment to treatment over the long term. It provides people a chance to more fully understand what treatment will reasonably involve and make a commitment accordingly. For example:

"Now that we've talked in some detail about your current crisis, the fact that you've been feeling suicidal for some time now, and that previous treatment efforts have not been particularly successful, I would like to ask you to make a commitment to coming in for three additional sessions in order to complete an extended evaluation. This will give me the opportunity to understand your history better, come to a more accurate diagnosis, and offer sound recommendations about what treatment approach I believe most appropriate. It will give you a chance to get to know me better, to understand the treatment approach I use, what's expected of you in terms of time and homework, and make a decision as to whether or not you think this particular treatment approach will be helpful. If this sounds agreeable, then at the end of the fourth session you and I can come to some agreement as to whether or not you would like to continue in treatment. At that point, we can identify the goals for treatment and speculate about how long treatment will most likely last. If you're also seeing a psychiatrist, this will give me a chance to talk with your psychiatrist if you'd like and coordinate your care as much as possible."

Similarly the use of a treatment log can be introduced in the first session. For example:

"I believe it's important for you to keep a record of your treatment for use after you finish. That way, you can use what you've learned later on, particularly when it's needed. I also think it's important that you keep record of any conclusions you come to in the treatment process, including beliefs about yourself, others, and your future. As you'll discover as treatment progresses, you may also find that your beliefs about how you handle feelings, whether or not you can tolerate emotional pain, and other day-to-day skills may change considerably. Why don't we start with what you've concluded today. Have you come to any conclusions about anything in particular in the time that we've talked today? You've agreed to schedule at least three additional sessions and you sound a bit more hopeful. Also, you rated your emotional upset as having been reduced considerably in the brief time we've spent here today. Actually, we didn't have to do too much to diffuse the crisis. All we've done so far is talk and do a little problem solving. Does this tell you anything about your ability to tolerate and handle emotional pain or solve problems? Here's some paper, let's jot down and keep record of what you're thinking. I'll write today's date on this page so we can keep track of how things progress from week to week. Keeping a log like this should only take a few minutes each day."

Although Ms. D did not have any family available, the idea of interviewing and integrating family into the treatment process should be introduced in the first session. It is helpful to do so in an effort to get a more accurate picture of risk (i.e., objective markers of risk) as well as to implement any needed monitoring in between sessions. Undoubtedly, there will be circumstances in which integrating family would be inappropriate. For example, when family members are directly involved in the conflict or the crisis that precipitated the suicide attempt, when family members are emotionally unstable or otherwise impaired, when the patient refuses to allow their involvement, or when there is violence in the home, it would be best not to attempt active family involvement. Again, the idea of family involvement can be presented in a non-threatening manner. For example:

"If agreeable, I'd like to interview your husband. You've mentioned that the two of you have a supportive relationship, he brought you in today, and he's very concerned about your well-being. This will basically serve three purposes. First, it will provide me with additional information that will help me better understand your current situation and, as a result, variables that are important in assessing risk. Second, it might prove helpful in coordinating efforts to monitor how you're doing over the coming week prior to your next session. Between the three of us, I'm sure we can establish a schedule in which you won't spend time alone for several days. You mentioned that you're scared right now and don't want to be alone. Finally, it will help us determine what, if any, role your husband should play in the treatment process. What are your thoughts about this idea? Does it sound like having him involved in some fashion might be productive?"

As discussed in detail in Chapter 7, the need to articulate a crisis response plan is critical. By the end of the first session, you should have something down in writing. Ideally, the plan should be put on a piece of paper, on a 3 × 5 card, or on the back of a business card: anything that can be carried in a purse or wallet and easily accessed during a period of crisis. The need for a crisis response plan can be introduced in the following manner:

> "It sounds as though we both agree that things can be managed on an outpatient basis without the need for hospitalization. However, I'd like to make sure that we have an agreeable crisis response plan in place if a problem should surface in between sessions. As you've emphasized today, you've had difficulty thinking clearly when you get acutely upset. Why don't we review some of the things we've talked about and put them into a step-by-step plan that you can use if a crisis occurs? Let's write them down so that you can carry the plan with you and access it as needed. Here's a 3 × 5 card, that way you can just put the card in your purse, pull it out, and read it when there's a problem."

Session 1 lays the foundation for the rest of treatment. The clinician will have established a number of important expectations. First, the patient will assume considerable responsibility in the management of his or her suicidality. The crisis response plan is just one example; maintaining an active treatment log is another. Actually, this was something to which Ms. D responded quite favorably and found to be one of the more attractive aspects of the treatment model. Second, the importance of a collaborative approach is clear. Third, the central role of cognitive restructuring has been emphasized, although the ICARE model (see Chapter 8, this volume) has yet to be presented. Beliefs that comprise the suicidal belief system are being articulated, documented, and challenged from the very first session. Finally, the need for structure and planning in the treatment process are being communicated, both of which facilitate skill building that cut across the areas of self-monitoring, emotion regulation, and problem solving in particular.

Session 2 Agenda

Sessions 2 to 4 provide an opportunity to accomplish the remaining tasks mentioned in Chapter 5 and allow clinician and patient to come to some agreement about continuing care. In addition, for those patients for whom it is necessary, the clinician can initiate psychiatric care and psychotropic medication. It also provides the clinician an opportunity to access professional consultation if needed. Particularly for those patients with complex histories, considerable comorbidity, and chronic suicidality, it allows the clinician time to generate a more accurate conceptualization and to make meaningful estimates about the likely duration of treatment. Consistent with

a CBT orientation, each session should start with a brief review of any assigned homework and a discussion of the session agenda. For Session 2, the
agenda includes the following:

- Assess risk.
- Review homework (e.g., treatment log) and present the agenda for the
session.
- Complete the review of the patient's history of suicidal behavior and
prior treatment efforts, identifying what worked and what did not. It is important to get an accurate understanding of why previous treatment efforts failed.
Was the patient not adequately motivated? Did the patient not have the resources, financial or otherwise, to continue in treatment? Was there family op-
position or a lack of family support? Identifying these problems up front will
improve the likelihood that they can be effectively resolved.
- Determine baseline level of functioning including both direct and indirect markers of suicidality. Summarize baseline functioning using the summary sheets offered in Chapter 5. This will provide the clinician with markers
against which treatment progress can be gauged.
- Assign initial phase and level designations using the summary sheets
offered in Chapter 3. Again, this provides a means to gauge progress but also
to clearly communicate what is being targeted in treatment.
- Determine treatment targets in terms of prominent symptoms, deficient skills, and maladaptive personality traits.
- Continue to target symptom management and diffusing the suicidal
crisis as noted for Session 1.
- Review and document conclusions for the session in the patient's treatment log, emphasizing the patient's suicidal belief system. Also, have the patient write a brief three- or four-sentence summary of what was accomplished
during the session.
- For homework, initiate self-monitoring using the STR and the suicidal
cycle.
- Continue use of the crisis response plan.

Ms. D was assigned Level I across each treatment component (symptom
management, skill building, and personality development). The most prominent and problematic symptoms included current depressive symptoms; suicidal ideation that was frequent, intense, and specific; binge drinking; anger;
hopelessness; and self-mutilatory behavior. Ms. D started on antidepressant
medication and initiated self-monitoring. The most troublesome skill deficits
included emotion regulation, distress tolerance, and anger management. She
responded well to keeping a treatment log and actually came to a few conclusions after the initial session, stating, "I really do want to live," and "I can take
more pain than I thought."

As evidenced earlier, many of the tasks that need to be accomplished for Session 2 are decisions made by the clinician about the patient's current level of functioning, and, therefore, they do not require session time. The primary interventions for Session 2 include introduction of the STR and describing the suicidal cycle.

> "As we've discussed, there is a connection between what happens, what you think about it, what you feel, and ultimately whether or not you make a suicide attempt. Several times, you've mentioned that you didn't really see any connection between these things. I'd like to ask you to complete this suicidal thought record over the course of the coming week. It's really pretty easy to do and probably won't take you any more than 10 or so minutes a day. If you look across the top of the STR, you'll see that it has a place for you to write down what happened that triggered your suicidal thoughts. Then there is a place for you to document what the specific suicidal thoughts were, as well as what you were feeling at the time and what you ended up doing. Also, as you'll notice, there is a place for you to rate the severity of your thoughts and feelings as well as document how long they lasted. It's important for you to complete the ratings for several reasons. Doing is part of learning to regulate your feelings better, but the ratings will also help you come up with evidence to counter some of the beliefs you mentioned last time we met and today. For example, you said, 'I can't tolerate the pain anymore' or 'The pain I feel will never stop or get any better.' As you've demonstrated today, the pain you felt was cut by half simply by talking for 45 minutes.
>
> "It's also important to complete the STR because it will help us identify what your suicidal cycle is. In other words, we'll be able to identify the predictable steps you go through when you become suicidal. This is important for many reasons but primarily because it helps us identify what we can do at each point of that cycle. Specifically, it helps identify the kinds of thoughts and beliefs we need to target, the disruptive emotions and physical symptoms, and finally the behaviors that are geared toward suicide."

Session 3 Agenda

Sessions 3 and 4 provide the clinician an opportunity to complete the remaining goals detailed in Chapter 5 while also continuing interventions in terms of symptom and crisis management and associated cognitive restructuring, as well as initial skill building. The agenda for Session 3 includes the following:

- Assess risk.
- Review homework and present the agenda for the session.
- Provide a CBT conceptual model for the patient's suicidality using the suicidal mode worksheet presented in Chapter 2.
- Provide a detailed rationale for treatment using the handout in Chapter 5 (Figure 5.5).
- Complete psychological testing if indicated.
- Review conclusions for the session and document. Have the patient write a brief three- or four-sentence summary of what was accomplished during the session.
- Assign continued self-monitoring as homework.

The most critical goal of the session is to present a meaningful conceptual model for treatment (the patient's suicidal mode) and provide an accompanying rationale. The clinician will have already spent two sessions with the patient. He or she will more fully understand the patient's history and previous problems in treatment, if any, and should have a more clear picture of the diagnostic complexity and chronicity presented. The clinician can use the suicidal mode worksheet presented in Chapter 2 and the patient's self-monitoring logs to detail a suicidal cycle that is evident when the suicidal mode is active.

For Ms. D, this cycle was fairly repetitive and clearly evident in her STRs. She had a predictable cycle that was almost uniformly triggered by perceived interpersonal rejection of some sort. In terms of her suicidal belief system, the three primary themes mentioned in Chapter 2 were all present, including beliefs that she *couldn't tolerate the emotional pain* (poor distress tolerance), that she was *worthless and not worthy of a relationship* (unlovability), and that she did not *have the skills to cope* (helplessness). In terms of prominent symptoms, she reported a mixture of both depression and anxiety. In terms of her behavioral responses, Ms. D reported consistently engaging in behavior that only facilitated her feelings of helplessness and reinforced her suicidal belief system. In addition, her behavior (substance abuse, self-mutilatory behavior, and uncontrolled expression of anger) only exacerbated physiological arousal and heightened her suicide risk. As a result of the clear suicidal cycle identified, Ms. D was able to see that the primary targets in treatment would not just be management of her symptoms but also identification of her underlying vulnerabilities, including deficient skills in distress tolerance, emotion regulation, and anger management, as well as her associated suicidal belief system. Any changes that occur in these areas are evidence of at least minimal personality development (consistent with the definition of personality psychopathology presented in DSM-IV). Also, Ms. D completed some psychological testing to assist in differential diagnosis and treatment planning. Specifically, she completed the Minnesota Multiphasic Personality Inventory-2 and the Millon Clinical Multiaxial Inventory-III.

The conceptual model can be presented in straightforward language. For example:

"Let's talk in a little more detail about what leads to your suicidal behavior and also make it a little more clear what it is we're trying to accomplish in treatment. As I've mentioned before, there are three different parts that we're going to be targeting. We're going to target not only your symptoms of depression and anxiety but also your beliefs about killing yourself and what it is that you do in an effort to cope with feeling this way. Let's map out an example. As you've mentioned on your STRs, you have a range of thoughts about killing yourself when you feel criticized or rejected by your husband. This is the triggering event; it's an external event. At other times, you've mentioned being triggered by internal events such as having thoughts and images about the early abuse you suffered as a child. Once triggered, you've mentioned pretty consistent thoughts about suicide. It's important to recognize that not only have you had thoughts about suicide but that you've consistently mentioned thoughts about why you wanted to kill yourself. You've mentioned that you wanted to kill yourself because you didn't deserve to live, that you couldn't tolerate the feelings of pain, and that you were helpless to do anything about the way you've felt. This is one of the primary things we're going to target, the beliefs that you have about suicide and why you need to kill yourself. Once you start thinking about suicide, you've mentioned that your depression and anxiety intensify, that you notice physical symptoms including racing heart, increased respiration rate, mild sweating, muscle tension, and considerable anger and agitation. Ultimately, you've mentioned that you start drinking, at times lose control, break and throw things, call and yell at your husband, and sometimes cut on yourself. Finally, you mentioned that none of these things help and usually just make the problem worse. Actually, you've consistently said that when you act this way, you feel only more helpless and out of control. These are the other things we're going to target, helping you do things to relieve your anxiety and agitation and stop doing things that just tend to make you feel worse and increase the likelihood that you'll do something to hurt yourself. In other words, we're going to intervene in these three spots, with what you think, what you do to manage your feelings, and by attempting to reduce and eliminate the things you do that only prove to be self-destructive and self-defeating."

At the end of the session, when reviewing and documenting the patient's conclusions, it is important to start to organize them around the themes of the suicidal belief system, identified in Chapter 2. Specifically, the therapist can organize the patient's beliefs and pursue cognitive restructuring around the primary themes of unlovability, helplessness, and poor distress tolerance. For example:

> "Let's start to organize the conclusions that you've come to at the end of each session. As we've discussed before, there were a number of beliefs that you mentioned when you've been suicidal. Among them, you mentioned feeling worthless, helpless and like you couldn't tolerate or cope with the way you feel. It sounds like you've started to come to some conclusions that contradict those beliefs."

Session 4 Agenda

The primary agenda items for session 4 are to conclude the extended evaluation, review the rationale for treatment, and come to some agreement as to whether the patient will continue in therapy. In addition, it is important to offer some estimate as to the treatment time line. How long will treatment likely take and what can be accomplished? Finally, it is critical to spend a few minutes discussing the therapeutic alliance. Has an adequate working relationship been established? If not, what problems are evident? Devoting time to discussing the therapeutic relationship acknowledges and reinforces the idea that a healthy working alliance is critical to treatment success. The agenda for Session 4 includes the following:

- Assess risk.
- Review homework and present the agenda for the session.
- Complete the informed consent process using the handout provided in Chapter 5 and articulate an agenda for ongoing treatment.
- Identify and agree on treatment goals.
- Discuss the therapeutic alliance and any related problems.
- Review conclusions for the session and document in the treatment log. Have the patient write a brief three- or four-sentence summary of what was accomplished during the session.

Ms. D was agreeable to continuing in treatment and expressed few reservations about the process. Actually, she was encouraged by the commonsense nature of treatment to date and the *understandable model* that was presented. Moreover, she was very positive about the therapeutic alliance, noting that she felt like an *active partner in treatment*, perhaps for the first time. Previous problems in treatment were discussed in detail, the majority revolving around poor motivation and the belief that *things would not change.* As evident, considerable cognitive restructuring had already taken place by the end of the fourth session. Implicit in Ms. D's responses are hope and some optimism. All these beliefs and conclusions were documented in the patient's treatment log, suggestive of an evolving suicidal belief system.

Informed consent needs to be completed in as straightforward a manner as possible, preferably using the handout provided in Chapter 5. For example:

> "Now that we've completed the agreed upon number of sessions required for a thorough evaluation, it's important for us to come to some agreement as to whether or not you would like to continue in treatment, how long that might take, and what we might reasonably expect to accomplish. Remember that over the last two sessions we've talked about a conceptual model that would explain why you've become suicidal and what the underlying problems might be. Now let's review a few things about treatment and what we're trying to accomplish. [Figure 5.5 in Chapter 5 can then be reviewed.] In terms of the duration of treatment, in many ways, it will depend on how much you'd like to accomplish. As you've recognized in just the last few sessions, there is a belief system that helps maintain your suicidal behavior. You've already taken some significant steps to changing that belief system and developing some of the fundamental skills necessary to cope with stress and problems more effectively. There are, however, other problems that have been more chronic in nature including your problems with depression and posttraumatic stress disorder. These may take considerably more time to address. It is difficult to provide you with a definitive time line, but what we might want to do is agree on a set of goals for the next 5 months and then reevaluate your progress at that point. Then, if necessary, we can repeat the process and plan for 6-month blocks. How does this sound to you?"

For Ms. D, treatment goals were relatively straightforward and were summarized under each of the treatment components listed in the original case description. Given the chronic nature of her suicidality, 6-month blocks were used and her progress was reevaluated and new goals established accordingly.

Sessions 5–10: Symptom Management, Cognitive Restructuring, Reducing and Eliminating Suicidal Behaviors

For the next six sessions, the primary focus should revolve around continued symptom management, cognitive restructuring, and the reduction of any persistent suicidal or self-mutilatory behaviors. Cognitive restructuring (see Chapter 9, this volume) should be introduced through use of the ICARE model (ICARE is an acronym standing for the model's five steps: Identify, Connect, Assess, Restructure, and Execute). The symptom matching hierarchy can be modified as needed, and the hierarchy of core beliefs (discussed in Chapter 9, this volume) should be used to help keep track of changes in the suicidal belief system. As discussed in Chapter 8 (this volume), suicidal and self-mutilatory behaviors are reduced by the use of interventions that target the suicidal cycle in its earlier phases. This is generally consistent with evolving problem solving, emotion regulation, and distress tolerance skills (see Chapter 10, this volume). Accordingly, the crisis response plan will need to be periodically modified as skills develop. For the most part, the agenda for each of these sessions is comparable and will include the following:

- Assess risk.
- Review homework and present the agenda for the session.
- Establish a symptom matching hierarchy for targeted symptoms.
- Clearly articulate the suicidal cycle and identify target suicidal and self-destructive behaviors that need to be eliminated.
- Introduce the ICARE model for cognitive restructuring.
- Establish intervention plans for the early and late phase suicidal cycle. Introduce the crisis response plan first which targets the late phase of the suicidal cycle. Once the crisis plan is successfully implemented, interventions can address the suicidal cycle in its early phases.
- The patient's *philosophy-for-living statement* needs to started and modified periodically (see Chapter 9).
- Assign self-monitoring homework continuing to use the STR.
- Review conclusions for the session and document in the treatment log. Have the patient write a brief three- or four-sentence summary of what was accomplished during the session.

The agenda for sessions 5 through 10 will revolve primarily around symptom management and cognitive restructuring. The ICARE model should be introduced, emphasized, and used in fairly repetitive fashion. As progress is demonstrated, the idea of early-phase interventions should be introduced and emphasized, easing the transition to focusing more specifically on skill building for sessions 10 through 18. Early-phase intervention is basically a demonstration of new skills and can take the form of any of the skill-building targets (i.e., problem solving, anger management, assertiveness, distress tolerance, emotion regulation, or self-monitoring).

The ICARE model can be introduced in the following manner:

> "I would like to introduce a standard and simple approach to cognitive restructuring that you can use in any situation. It's easy to remember. Take a look at this sheet of paper [using the following list, the expanded STR in Figure 9.3, and the list of distortions in Figure 9.4]. As indicated, there are five steps I'd like you to go through each time you have a suicidal thought, let's start with number one and review and discuss each.

> "1. *Identify.* Identify the specific automatic thought and the underlying core belief. Write the thought/belief down on the expanded STR.
> "2. *Connect* the automatic thought to the distortion. Identify the distortion inherent to the belief.
> "3. *Assess* (evaluate) the thought/belief. What is the evidence for/against the belief? Are there other possible reasons/explanations for the situation/circumstance? What is the worst thing that could happen? The best? The most likely? Will it matter in a year?
> "4. *Restructure.* Restate the belief after having effectively evaluated it. What is a more reasonable alternative belief once the distortion has been removed and the belief decatastrophized? What are the advantages of giving up the dysfunctional suicidal belief identified?
> "5. *Execute* (respond). Act as though the new belief were true. Choose a behavior consistent with the new belief."

Just as with the ICARE model, the patient's need for a new *philosophy for living* needs to be introduced. This is a statement that summarizes new rules and assumptions for living. It can be kept as a part of the treatment log. It needs to be updated and modified periodically as changes occur in the suicidal belief system.

> "As we've discussed since our first session, it's important for you to develop a philosophy for living rather than one geared toward suicide. Along these lines, I'd like for you to keep track of those beliefs in your treatment log that are more consistent with this idea. In other words, I'd like for you to keep track of those beliefs that make it eas-

ier for you to live day to day, that are more reasonable and compassionate. For example, let's make a list of a few beliefs you've mentioned over the past few sessions:

"1.   Accept the fact that I'm not perfect and never will be.
"2.   Do the best job I can and feel good about it.
"3.   Recognize the things I do well each and every day.
"4.   Identify and work on accepting the things I cannot change, in myself, others, and the world around me.
"5.   Accept the fact that bad things are going to happen to me and I need to learn to deal better with them when they do."

Ms. D had little difficulty during this stage of treatment, responding well and expressing considerable motivation. Her symptoms remitted within a few weeks, responding well to both medication and activities geared toward specific symptoms from the symptom matching hierarchy. She made frequent and consistent use of the ICARE model for cognitive restructuring, evidencing considerable change in her suicidal belief system over a matter of just a few weeks. Actually, she commented on several occasions that she could not believe that she thought that way but was totally unaware of the beliefs or the repetitive cycle to her suicidality until we targeted each specifically. Finally, she developed a new philosophy for living and was able to implement it on a daily basis.

Sessions 10–19: Emphasis on Skill Building

Once the fundamentals of cognitive restructuring have been accomplished and symptoms have been well contained, the focus of treatment for Sessions 10 through 19 can shift more readily to deficient skills. Again, the agenda for each session can be much the same, with some variability depending on the particular skills being targeted. The skills can be targeted in variable order, depending on those identified as deficient through use of a skill deficiency hierarchy. Chapter 10 provides an example of one such hierarchy. The particular skills targeted during Sessions 10 through 19 are entirely dependent on the needs of the individual patient. It is important to be flexible here and target those skills first that are determined to be most important. As discussed in Chapter 10, a range of techniques can be used during these sessions including role play, behavioral rehearsal, and videotaping with review and feedback, as well as occasional *in vivo* exercises. It is important to use fairly simple and straightforward approaches to skills training consistent with those approaches offered in Chapter 10. We strongly recommend the liberal use of coping cards as a reminder. We have found coping cards to be an indispensable part of treatment. Patients find them understandable, respond well to them, and make consistent use of the cards. The cards facilitate the notion of *skill development homework*. In other words, we assign use of the card for the coming week as homework, along with continued self-monitoring using the STR. This amounts to early-phase intervention and further undermines the potential for any reemergence of suicidality. For the skills training sessions, we recommend the following agenda:

- Assess risk.
- Review homework and present the agenda for the session.
- Establish a skill deficiency hierarchy.
- Focus on a targeted skill.
- Assign skill development homework.
- Review conclusions for the session and document them in the treatment log. Have the patient write a brief three- or four-sentence summary of what was accomplished during the session.

The transition to skill building is an easy one, making good sense in terms of the conceptual model being used. Skill building can be introduced in the following manner:

"For the next ten sessions, I'd like for us to shift focus a bit and target those skills that we've identified as creating problems for you. From your hierarchy, it looks like interpersonal assertiveness and anger management are particular problems. What I'd like for us to do is to continue with our work on changing your suicidal belief system as well as continuing to complete the STRs, but also work directly on these two skill areas. If you look back at the suicidal cycle that we outlined, the idea is that these two problem areas likely created some of the vulnerability that triggered your suicidal thoughts to begin with. In other words, we'll be targeting things that we believe are likely causes of your suicidality. How does this sound to you?"

As with other aspects of treatment, Ms. D did well with focused skill building. She targeted primarily basic self-monitoring skills, emotion regulation, distress tolerance, and anger management. We made use of frequent role playing, supplemented with videotaping. It is important to remember that as skills develop, the patient's suicidal belief system will continue to evolve. This was the case with Ms. D, who proudly responded after a few sessions, "I can do a lot more things than I thought!" The change evident in this simple statement is considerable. Not only is it a sign of hopefulness, but it also gives us a glimpse of an emerging self-image that is markedly more positive, accompanied by a new found sense of efficacy.

Sessions 19–20: A Shift toward Personality Development and Longer-Term Treatment

Although personality development is something that is being addressed throughout treatment, the importance of targeting early developmental trauma and related self-image and interpersonal issues can be emphasized later in treatment. At this point, a decision needs to be made about the availability or necessity of longer-term care. The cognitive restructuring and skill development already accomplished has, by definition, resulted in some personality change. Sessions 19 and 20 can be used to discuss the nature of personality psychopathology and the likelihood that it will require longer-term care. If treatment is continued, many of the cognitive restructuring and skill-building tasks discussed earlier will be continued and emphasized from time to time but are likely to be supplemented by other CBT approaches for specific problems (e.g., cognitive processing therapy for posttraumatic stress disorder).

The need for ongoing therapy is best determined by the following factors: (1) the chronicity of the patient's suicidal behavior, (2) the patient's Axis I and II comorbidity, (3) the strengths identified in treatment so far, (4) the patient's level for each treatment component, and (5) the patient's responsiveness to both medication and psychotherapy. The need for longer-term care is always an individual clinical decision. However, the time-limited approach presented here will certainly help clinicians identify specific problem areas and treatment targets and negotiate (if needed) for additional coverage.

> "As you'll recall, we talked about completing 20 sessions and then reevaluating your progress and discussing the need for any ongoing treatment. Let's review what you've accomplished to date. Why don't you take out your treatment log and let's go through it. [The log is reviewed.] Clearly, you've accomplished an enormous amount. You've not had suicidal thoughts in quite some time, you've learned a number of new skills, and used them on a regular basis when you've been stressed. However, we've also talked about the fact that you've struggled with the memories of past sexual and physical abuse for some time now. This might be an opportunity to spend time on those issues specifically, now that you've effectively built some skills and resolved the recurrent suicidal crises. Let's talk a little about the advantages and disadvantages of continuing in treatment. If you decide that you'd like to continue, we need to be very specific about goals.

If treatment is discontinued, it is important to clearly document the progress made. This can be done in fairly simple fashion by noting (1) the patient's level accomplished for each treatment component, (2) the risk category and severity rating at the end of treatment, (3) direct and indirect markers of suicidality using the summary sheet provided earlier, (4) the changes evident in the patient's suicidal belief system, (5) new skills developed, (6) remission of targeted symptoms, and (7) personality changes implicit in the foregoing.

This chapter has provided session-by-session guidelines for a time-limited course of treatment. In the chapters that now follow, we discuss in detail specific procedures for evaluation and treatment.

5

The Evaluation Process and the Initial Interviews

In all clinical environments, the initial evaluation, including the initial interview, is critical to establishing a solid foundation for ongoing treatment, both short and long term. This is particularly true for those presenting with suicidality, a fact only magnified by time constraints. This chapter discusses the structure and goals of the evaluation process which may take anywhere from one to four sessions, depending on the complexity, severity, and chronicity of the individual presenting for treatment. Rice and Jobes (1997) and Rudd, Joiner, Jobes, and King (1999) have recommended that clinicians negotiate an *extended evaluation* period for suicidal patients with a goal of making a preliminary set of treatment recommendations *only after* thorough evaluation.

The goal of this extended evaluation is for the clinician to make a preliminary set of recommendations about the best course of care for the patient, and for the patient to thereby determine his or her best choices as to how to proceed. For example, the clinician may recommend treatment elsewhere in a different clinical setting or with another clinician if that is in the patient's best interest. The patient, in turn, may agree or disagree with the clinician's recommendations but either way is free to choose how to proceed. In many cases, the best option is to contract for a specific period (e.g., three to four sessions). This approach then provides yet a second opportunity at the end of the contracted period for the clinician to make further treatment recommendations from a more knowledgeable perspective and for the patient to then choose his or her best course of care. It is important to note that providing thorough informed consent from the start creates a shared understanding of the *ground rules* of treatment. We offer more about this later in the chapter. In that regard the imminently suicidal patient does not have to be surprised that inpatient hospitalization may be the recommendation and the necessary intervention of choice for the clinician. But short of the clear-and-imminent danger threshold, there is considerable room for both parties to evaluate and discern the most viable course of outpatient treatment.

The advantages of an *extended evaluation* are many, but perhaps most important:

1. It provides the clinician adequate time to come to a fairly accurate working diagnosis (both Axis I and II).
2. It allows for a more detailed and thorough understanding of those factors related to the patient's suicidality.
3. It allows the clinician to establish an initial risk level and estimate current level of functioning.
4. It provides an opportunity to develop a working conceptual model for treatment, that is, to complete the suicidal mode.
5. It provides an opportunity to establish adequate rapport.
6. It allows the clinician an opportunity to observe the patient over at least a limited period, something particularly important for chronically suicidal patients.

In short, the initial interview will undoubtedly vary in duration from patient to patient, but its structure and identifiable goals should be consistent across all cases. Occasionally, a single session will be adequate for a first-time attempter who has no prior history and a clear and uncomplicated diagnostic picture (i.e., no significant comorbidity). To be thorough and to accomplish the goals identified, however, clinicians should expect to need more than a single session and most frequently two to three. This is particularly true when it comes to delineating a meaningful conceptual model for the chronic multiple attempter, requiring a detailed understanding of prior attempts and their context. As noted in Chapter 3 (this volume), the treatment plan relies on an accurate conceptualization of the suicidal mode plus an understanding of severity, chronicity, and diagnostic complexity.

This chapter focuses specifically on issues related to suicidality. It is assumed that a thorough and complete intake history and diagnostic interview are completed for all patients and an initial diagnosis determined, regardless of the clinical presentation. As a result, these issues are not covered. They are assumed to be part of the *basic skills* inherent to clinical practice. It is assumed that a *standard clinical interview* includes at a minimum:

- General descriptive information (marital status, current living and work situations, age, etc.).
- Personal and social history including family, educational, and developmental history.
- A description of presenting problems including identifiable stressors and symptoms (i.e., to include onset, duration, and comorbidity) consistent with a diagnostic interview in accordance with DSM-IV necessary for differential diagnosis.
- Psychiatric and treatment history.
- Review of current supportive resources and interpersonal relationships.
- Related medical history and physical problems.
- Expectations regarding therapy and the treatment process.

In terms of suicidality, the goals for the initial interview(s) fall into four distinct categories, each critical to establishing a solid foundation for ongoing treatment:

1. Risk assessment.
2. Treatment conceptualization and consent.
3. Consultation and psychological testing.
4. The therapeutic relationship.

Each of these areas is discussed in more detail later, along with a clinical example. A section is also included that addresses the role of formal psychological testing and the use of psychometric instruments in the assessment and treatment process. As has been emphasized in previous chapters, the time constraints frequently experienced in treating suicidality in today's mental health marketplace demand an organized and efficient approach. The interview structure provided results in data useful in negotiating for longer-term care, if necessary, with the insurance carrier or case manager. We have found nothing more convincing than solid, understandable, and clinically relevant data, particularly when it is specific as to recurrent and potentially lethal attempts. We have yet to have a case manager deny some form of continuing care for a patient with precise and thorough documentation of chronic high risk with acute exacerbation (see Chapter 6).

In addition to the standard clinical interview, there are 13 tasks unique to the assessment of suicidality. They can be organized within the four broad categories identified previously (see Table 5.1) and need to be completed during the initial extended evaluation period:

TABLE 5.1. Goals for the Initial Evaluation Interview(s)

Category	Goal(s):
I: Risk assessment	1. Complete a thorough history of suicidality. 2. Assign initial risk category and risk severity ratings. 3. Interview family members, significant other(s) to assist in the above tasks, if available.
II: Treatment conceptualization and consent	1. Provide a CBT conceptual model (the suicidal mode) of the patient's suicidality to the patient. 2. Determine baseline level of functioning (i.e., direct and indirect markers of suicidality). 3. Assign initial phase and level designations. 4. Determine corresponding treatment targets. 5. Provide a detailed rationale for treatment, with goals and process to be followed. 6. Complete the informed consent process, providing written documentation for the patient. 7. Initiate self-monitoring.
III: Consultation and psychological testing	1. Complete initial psychological testing. 2. Access any needed consultation, psychiatric or otherwise.
IV: The therapeutic relationship	1. Establish the foundation for a productive working relationship and strong therapeutic relationship. 2. Define role of family members (if any) in treatment process.

1. Complete a thorough history of suicidality—including ideation, attempts, and related behaviors—detailing outcome and related medical and psychiatric care, as well as the full range of contextual variables identified in Chapter 6.
2. Determine the current frequency and severity of ideation, attempts, and related self-destructive or self-mutilatory behaviors.
3. Assign an initial risk category and risk severity rating (see Chapter 6).
4. Assign initial treatment component and level designations in accordance with current symptomatology and level of functioning (see Chapter 3).
5. Identify corresponding treatment targets.
6. Provide a CBT *conceptual model* of the patient's suicidality; that is, the clinician should confirm his or her conceptualization of the suicidal mode with the patient and educate the patient about the nature of the problem (see Chapter 2).
7. Provide a corresponding rationale for treatment, identifying specific goals and the process to be followed.

8. Initiate self-monitoring (using suicidal thought records, treatment logs, journals).
9. Complete initial psychological testing.
10. Access any needed consultation, psychiatric or otherwise.
11. Establish the foundation for a productive working relationship and strong therapeutic alliance.
12. Interview family members and significant others routinely, defining their role (if any) in the treatment and assessment process.
13. Complete *informed consent* procedures, providing a copy of written documentation to the patient.

Risk Assessment Goals: The Importance of Establishing a Baseline for Ongoing Monitoring

Within the first of the four categories, risk assessment, there are three primary goals for the initial interview. First, a thorough history of suicidality needs to be completed. This can be done in accordance with the framework outlined in Chapter 6. The framework offers a detailed listing of both categories and relevant questions in order to complete a thorough history (i.e., Categories I-VIII; see Figure 6.2). Second, the patient needs to be assigned an initial risk category and risk severity rating. The importance of establishing a baseline for the patient cannot be overstated. Without establishing a baseline for risk and current functioning, progress will prove virtually impossible to monitor over time, the conceptual model will likely be inaccurate, and a potentially unstable foundation is established for ongoing treatment. Often, progress with chronically suicidal patients is manifest in subtle but nonetheless significant ways. It is not uncommon for a thorough history to uncover self-mutilatory and self-destructive behaviors that may not have been voluntarily offered otherwise. These behaviors are frequently the first to be eliminated (see Chapter 8). If they were to go undetected, significant markers of treatment success would be lost.

The final risk assessment goal is to interview family member(s) and significant other(s) to assist in the treatment and risk assessment process. Naturally, the patient's consent is necessary except in cases of acute, imminent suicidality. The role of family members and significant others in the assessment process has been discussed in considerable detail elsewhere (e.g., Clark & Fawcett, 1992). When interviewing family members the clinician needs to do the following:

• Educate family about suicide risk and communication by discussing with them relevant markers of suicide risk. In essence, the clinician wants to enlist the family members in the monitoring and risk assessment process by telling them what to look for and how to recognize them importance of potentially subtle behaviors.

• Gather external information that will aid in risk assessment by asking about any recent examples of suicidal ideation or behavior by the patient.

• Communicate to family members that interest in what they have to say. The clinician will need to review some of the constraints presented by confidentiality but also reinforce that during periods of acute suicide risk confidentiality becomes a secondary concern.

• Let family members know that they play a role in the treatment process. As mentioned in later chapters, the clinician will also need to discuss appropriate limits and boundaries in treatment. The clinician does not want family members *intruding* and disrupting treatment

• Take advantage of the opportunity to rally and organize the patient's social support system by routinely integrating family members into the treatment process during periods of heightened risk.

• Clearly define a role for family in the treatment process. Tell family members how often they can expect to be involved and in what capacity (e.g., occasional marital or family sessions). Chronic, multiple attempters can often be treated effectively on an outpatient basis if adequate support can be mustered. If their role is defined, it is often easier to enlist family members in treatment later on if necessary. For example, the need for family or marital therapy is not uncommon. If family members have been engaged from the beginning, subsequent marital or family therapy is often less threatening and much more productive.

Treatment Conceptualization and Consent: Setting the Stage

The majority of the tasks for the initial interview target treatment conceptualization and consent (see Table 5.1). Most clinicians would agree that suicidality is often characterized as chaotic, unpredictable, and anxiety provoking for both the patient and the clinician. Establishing organization and coherency to treatment from the outset has a calming effect, reducing peripheral dysphoria about *what to do, how to do it,* and *for how long.* Such structure allows the patient and the clinician to focus on the multiple tasks at hand (i.e., assessment and treatment).

Determining Baseline Level of Functioning

One of the first tasks the clinician needs to complete is determining the patient's baseline level of functioning (i.e., direct and indirect markers of suicidality). There are many ways to address current level of functioning. At the most conspicuous level, current functioning is determined by assessing the frequency, intensity (i.e., severity), and duration of suicidal thoughts and behaviors. As discussed in Chapter 6, it is critical to distinguish between suicidal (i.e., with associated intent to die) and self-destructive or self-mutilatory behaviors (e.g., self-cutting, burning, or other mutilating behaviors with no associated intent to die), regardless of whether or not both are being targeted. A patient can continue to engage in self-mutilation and by no means be suicidal. If the distinction is not made, the treatment process is often confounded and specific targets poorly defined.

We recommend that the clinician complete a frequency, intensity/severity, and duration count for suicidal thoughts, attempts, and related self-destructive or self-mutilatory behaviors (i.e., an indirect marker of suicidality; see Figure 5.1). For suicide attempts, we recommend that both frequency and lethality be monitored. Simple subjective reports are also recommended rather than frequent and repetitive use of assessment instruments for ideation or suicidality. However, instruments such as the Beck Scale for Suicide Ideation (self-report; Beck & Steer, 1993) and the Modified Scale for Suicidal Ideation (clinician-rated; Miller, Norman, Bishop, & Dow, 1986) are useful when accessed on a periodic basis, offering some objective data to bolster and counterbalance subjective report. Some of the reasons for this recommendation are discussed in a later section, along with a thorough review of available instruments.

Similarly, a severity rating should be completed for indirect markers, particularly symptoms such as depression, anxiety, and hopelessness. Other significant symptoms can be included depending on the individual clinical presentation (e.g., guilt, anger, shame, and anhedonia). We recommend use of standardized (but brief) symptom monitoring scales when at all possible. For example, the Beck Scales for depression (Beck, Steer, & Brown, 1996), anxiety (Beck & Steer, 1993), and hopelessness (Beck & Steer, 1988) are ideal. They were developed for this purpose and can be used with ease and provide a reliable and valid assessment of symptoms. When an assessment instrument is not available, the use of simple subjective ratings provides a means of monitoring change over time (see Chapter 6). Finally, we recommend that a simple summary rating be completed indicating *overall level of functioning*. Although this rating is highly subjective, it provides an integration of direct and indirect markers into a concise numeric rating for monitoring purposes. Given the broad and very general purpose of the rating, the following range is suggested: 1–3 (mild impairment), 4–7 (moderate impairment), 8–10 (severe impairment).

Figure 5.1 provides a summary sheet for both direct and indirect markers of suicidality. The clinician can simply copy the sheet and use it as an organizational tool. It is particularly useful because it summarizes the relevant data on a single page that can be inserted into the clinical chart, supplementing rou-

Patient name: _____

Direct markers of suicidality

Suicidal thoughts:	Frequency	Daily _____
		Weekly _____
		Monthly _____
	Severity rating (1–10) _____	
	Duration (sec/min/hr) _____	
	Specificity rating (1–10) _____	

Suicide attempts   Frequency _____
                       (i.e., since starting treatment)
                       Lethality rating (1–10) _____
                       (i.e., for last attempt)

Beck Scale for Suicide   Score
Ideation   Initial _____
                          Periodic (Date:) _____
                          Termination _____

Indirect markers of suicidality

Depression   BDI-II score   _____

Anxiety   BAI score   _____

Hopelessness   BHS score   _____

Other (e.g., guilt, anger)

Specify:

_____	Rating (1–10)	_____
_____	Rating (1–10)	_____
_____	Rating (1–10)	_____
_____	Rating (1–10)	_____

Other self-destructive, self-mutilatory behaviors (specify)

_____	Frequency	_____
_____	(indicate weekly, monthly)	_____
_____		_____

Overall level of   Rating (1–10)   _____
functioning

FIGURE 5.1. Summary of ratings for direct and indirect markers of suicidality. From *Treating Suicidal Behavior: An Effective, Time-Limited Approach* by M. David Rudd, Thomas Joiner, and M. Hasan Rajab. Copyright 2001 by The Guilford Press. Permission to reproduce this figure is granted to purchasers of this book for personal use only (see copyright page for details).

tine clinical entries. We recommend the use of the summary sheet with regularity (e.g., daily or weekly during periods of heightened or acute risk and less frequently as risk diminishes, perhaps monthly).

Figure 5.2 provides an example of a completed form for Ms. D, the case described in Chapter 4. The specific information provided in the rating summary about Ms. D's direct and indirect markers of suicidality clearly delineate her *moderate–severe impairment* status (i.e., overall level of functioning). Although she presents with considerable severity and chronicity, direct markers of suicidality do not reveal any imminent risk, supporting the feasibility of outpatient treatment. She noted specific ideation (i.e., *shooting herself*), reported that they were only fleeting thoughts (despite high frequency), and, most important, voiced no stated intent or prepatory behaviors whatsoever. In contrast to routine clinical chart entries, the summary of ratings provided in Figure 5.2 offers an easily accessible distillation of information critical to clinical decision making. As illustrated, a thorough review of baseline level of functioning during the initial interview provides a means to monitor treatment progress (or decline) in a consistent and comprehensive fashion.

Assigning Initial Phase and Level and Treatment Targets

After determining baseline level of functioning, it is necessary to assign initial phase and level designations for treatment. Ms. D was assigned the following phase and level designations: crisis phase, Level I (stabilization); skill-building phase, Level I (acquisition); and personality development phase, Level I (stabilization). These allow the clinician to determine corresponding treatment targets and have an initial treatment plan.

INITIAL TREATMENT PLAN

Symptom Management Component, Level I (Stabilization). The patient is not currently capable of managing her suicidal crises without external assistance and intervention. The patient's suicidality is a chronic problem and she has never developed adequate skills to manage these recurrent crises on her own. She has always relied on external resources, be it family, friends, or a clinician. Accordingly, initial efforts would be characterized by symptom management and related crisis intervention tasks with a focus on specific symptomatology, including (1) remission of depressive symptoms, (2) reduced suicidality (ideation frequency, specificity, intent), (3) resolution of acute anger, hopelessness, (4) elimination of binge drinking, and (5) elimination of self-mutilatory behavior. In addition to psychotherapy, medication would likely be effective and a necessary component of treatment assisting with symptom remission. Accordingly, referral to a psychiatrist would be indicated.

Patient name: <u>Ms. D</u>

Direct markers of suicidality

Suicidal thoughts:	Frequency	Daily <u>10x</u>
		Weekly _____
		Monthly _____
	Severity rating (1–10) <u>9</u>	
	Duration (sec/min/hr) <u>2–3 seconds</u>	
	Specificity rating (1–10) <u>7</u>	

Suicide attempts   Frequency <u>Not applicable</u>
(i.e., since starting treatment)
Lethality rating (1–10) <u>Not applicable</u>
(i.e., for last attempt)

Beck Scale for Suicide   Score
Ideation   Initial <u>18</u>
   Periodic (Date:) _____
   Termination _____

Indirect markers of suicidality

Depression	BDI-II score	<u>32—severe</u>
Anxiety	BAI score	<u>17—moderate</u>
Hopelessness	BHS score	<u>11—moderate</u>

Other (e.g., guilt, anger)

Specify:

<u>Anger</u>	Rating (1–10)	<u>8</u>
<u>Guilt</u>	Rating (1–10)	<u>8</u>
<u>Shame</u>	Rating (1–10)	<u>7</u>
_____	Rating (1–10)	_____

Other self-destructive, self-mutilatory behaviors (specify)

<u>Self-cutting</u>	Frequency	<u>2 × monthly</u>
<u>Binge drinking</u>	(indicate weekly, monthly)	<u>2 × monthly</u>
_____		_____

| **Overall level of functioning** | Rating (1–10) | <u>8—moderate–severe impairment</u> |

FIGURE 5.2. Example of a completed summary of ratings for direct and indirect markers of suicidality.

Skill-Building Component, Level I (Acquisition). The patient possesses minimal skills and would require comprehensive skill training and development, but initial efforts would focus on improved self-monitoring, emotion regulation, distress tolerance, and anger management.

Personality Development Component, Level I (Stabilization). The patient would require stabilization of recurrent and severe crises in order to focus on skill acquisition and enduring changes in long-standing maladaptive personality traits. Personality components that would naturally be woven into ongoing interventions would include (1) image of self as defective, (2) perception of others as rejecting and abandoning, and (3) resolution of childhood sexual abuse (posttraumatic stress disorder symptoms, feelings of guilt shame, and excessive responsibility).

As the case of Ms. D illustrates, the initial treatment plan for someone manifesting recurrent and chronic suicidality is relatively broad in nature. Paradoxically, however, the focus of the treatment is specific given that we have used the treatment matrix to target specific skills and personality components. In a managed care environment, it is essential that we discuss in a specific and conceptually meaningful way what we are doing in psychotherapy, one that is readily understandable from provider to provider not just those applying the same theoretical model. In general, Ms. D's suicidal mode has a low threshold and is easily triggered. Even during periods of relative calm, it is likely that there are a number of facilitating modes that complicate the clinical landscape. Despite the clinical complexity inherent to someone with chronic suicidality, the treatment-planning matrix translates the web of potential treatment issues into a concise list easily understood by clinician, patients, and insurance administrators.

Outlining the Suicidal Mode

Completing the steps summarized earlier should allow the clinician to begin the process of articulating a CBT conceptual model of the patient's suicidality (i.e., the suicidal mode consistent with the framework provided in Chapter 2). To do so, we need to identify predisposing vulnerabilities and identifiable triggers, as well as define the structural content of the cognitive, affective, physiological and behavioral systems. The suicidal mode summary worksheet introduced in Chapter 2 can be used in this process. Figure 5.3 is an example of Ms. D's worksheet. Figure 5.4 provides a simple conceptual model of the *suicidal mode* for Ms. D This conceptual model is useful in talking with the patient about the nature of suicidal crises, how we understand them theoretically and in terms of applicable research, and ultimately what we actually do in

Patient name: Ms. D

Treatment point (circle one):   Intake assessment   <u>Completed on 7-1-98</u>

                                      Periodic review, No. of sessions ____

                                      Transition or referral _____

                                      Termination, planned _____

                                      Termination, unplanned (e.g., abrupt discontinuation)

Symptom management component (circle one):	Level I: Symptom stabilization (circled)
	Level II: Symptom self-management
	Level III: Symptom utilization

Current target(s):

Remission of depressive symptoms, reduced suicidality, i.e., reduced ideation frequency, specificity, intent. Resolution of acute anger, hopelessness. Eliminate binge drinking and self-mutilatory behavior.

Skill building component (circle one):	Level I: Skill acquisition (circled)
	Level II: Skill refinement
	Level III: Skill generalization

Current target(s):

Comprehensive skill training and development, starting with distress tolerance and emotion regulation.

Personality development (circle one):	Level I: Personality stabilization (circled)
	Level II: Personality modification
	Level III: Personality refinement

Current target(s):

Stabilize recurrent crises in order to focus on initial skill acquisition. Currently, personality dysfunction includes self-image as defective, perceptions of others as rejecting and abandoning, and chronic problems secondary to childhood sexual abuse.

Notes: *Referral for immediate medication consultation.*

FIGURE 5.3. Example of a completed treatment component and level worksheet.

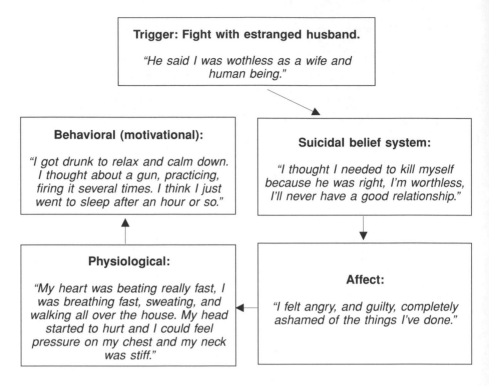

FIGURE 5.4. The suicidal mode for a single episode of suicidality: The case of Ms. D.

psychotherapeutic treatment. It is important that the model be simple, straight-forward, and understandable. Using direct quotes from the patient's STR (when available) is the most efficient and effective approach. Essentially, the conceptual model provides a springboard to discussing the rationale for treatment, particularly in terms of specific treatment targets and the process to be followed.

As illustrated in Figure 5.4, Ms. D's suicidal crises have been fairly consistent over time, routinely triggered by a conflict with her estranged spouse (or family members). Such a conflict triggered her suicidal belief system, which was dominated by thoughts of defectiveness, worthlessness, and hopelessness. She reported subsequent feelings of intense anger, shame, guilt, and depression. She described strong physiological arousal, and ultimately binge drinking and some limited prepatory behavior (i.e., getting her gun out). This brief model provides an understandable distillation of an enormous amount of information. When the model for Ms. D was completed and presented to her, Ms. D's response was as follows:

THERAPIST (*completing the drawing of the model*): Well, here's the model we identified for your last crisis. Does it look accurate; could you share your impressions?

MS. D: That's me! I can't believe we could put it down on paper like that. I feel like I kind of understand what the problem is, I hope I can change it!

We recommend that patients be given a written description of the treatment rationale. Figure 5.5 provides a sample statement that could be given to patients. It is important that it not be loaded with jargon or so detailed as to detract from the message that this problem is one that can be understood and changed. If a conceptual model for the problem is agreed on and the treatment rationale is discussed, necessary informed consent to treatment can be accomplished without marked difficulty.

Confidentiality and Informed Consent

Two additional goals are to be accomplished in the *treatment conceptualization and consent* category. They include completing the informed consent process and initiating self-monitoring (something that is also discussed in detail in the following chapters). The ethical guidelines of the American Psychological Association (1992) are explicit about the importance of providing appropriate and understandable informed consent to any patient seeking clinical treatment (Section 4.02), as well as the need for structuring the clinical relationship with the patient (Section 4.01). These ethical guidelines are certainly relevant across clinical presentations, but they are particularly critical to clinical work with suicidal patients. At a fundamental level, the potential life-and-death nature of the suicidal presentation creates an inherent paradox that can potentially strike at the heart of therapeutic work. To be specific, it is axiomatic that confidentiality is essential to building a strong therapeutic alliance, yet legal statutes in the United States typically *require* the breach of confidentiality in cases in which there is imminent physical danger to self or others. In cases of imminently suicidal patients, clinicians may breach patient confidentiality to ensure the physical safety of such patients (i.e., patients are placed into inpatient settings, whether or not they want to be). The clinician may be following legal requirements, but such interventions are not always welcomed by suicidal patients, who may feel coercively tricked, trapped, and otherwise disinclined to ever seek mental health treatment again (Szasz, 1986).

Thus, at a fundamental level, the life-and-death nature of suicidality can potentially pit patients (who may see suicide as a personal right) against their clinician (who may understand that preventing suicide, using whatever means necessary, is both a statutory and professional obligation). Unfortunately, the potential for an adversarial power struggle around issues of safety and hospi-

PURPOSE AND NATURE OF PROCEDURES

Mental health professionals help patients with mental or emotional difficulties such as depression or anxiety, family problems, adjustment difficulties, personality problems, or grief, among many others. You've been referred because of problems with suicidal thoughts and behaviors. To better understand you and your particular problems, you'll be asked to complete an extended evaluation, ranging from one to four sessions. This will involve a clinical interview, some psychological testing, and possibly consultation with other psychiatric, mental health, and/or medical professionals. You might be asked to talk to a psychiatrist about medication. We might also need to access your previous psychiatric/psychological records and possibly talk to family members or significant others. We want to make sure that we clarify your diagnosis, understand your specific problems, and make appropriate treatment recommendations.

ABOUT THIS TREATMENT

Suicidal behavior is thought to be the result of many different factors, including your developmental history (things that happened to you when you were growing up), formal psychiatric diagnoses (e.g., depression), and the way in which you deal with stress (such as the breakup of a marriage). The treatment that you are considering views suicide as the result of the way you think about and solve problems. One way that you've attempted to solve your problems is by considering suicide as an option. This is what we'd like to help you change.

Psychotherapy is a joint effort between the psychologist or mental health professional and you to alleviate the problems that brought you here. Your progress will depend on many factors such as the complexity of the problem, the skill of the treatment staff, your motivation and investment in treatment, and other life circumstances. Although results cannot be guaranteed, most patients find that they benefit in some way from therapy.

The therapy you are considering will target some very specific things. First, we'll try to help you reduce the intensity of such current symptoms as depression, anxiety, hopelessness, insomnia, or anger. In particular, we'll attempt to help you get a little better at tolerating your own feelings and responding in a healthier way. Medication might be an alternative if the symptoms are severe. We'll also work on very specific skills such as problem solving, emotion regulation (dealing better with your feelings), anger management, and assertiveness. Working on the way you think about things will be central to treatment. For example, you might have a tendency to be catastrophic, or to blow things out or proportion, when stressed. This is something we'll work on. Finally, we'll work on long-standing problems you've described with your self-image, such as believing you're a terrible person. As a part of this, you'll more than likely be asked to address any childhood trauma such as sexual or physical abuse.

Aside from this form of therapy, we currently offer other forms of individual or group psychotherapy, as well as medication. If you'd like to talk with someone else about other approaches, an appointment can be arranged.

You should expect to have some strong feelings in therapy. Therapy can result in individual change and unleash strong feelings. You should be aware of the possibility for potential emotional, family, or marital strain which may occur during treatment.

(continued)

FIGURE 5.5. Treatment rationale handout example. Some of the limitations on confidentiality (e.g., abuse reporting requirements) vary from state to state. From *Treating Suicidal Behavior: An Effective, Time-Limited Approach* by M. David Rudd, Thomas Joiner, and M. Hasan Rajab. Copyright 2001 by The Guilford Press. Permission to reproduce this figure is granted to purchasers of this book for personal use only (see copyright page for details).

Treatment frequency and duration will vary from individual to individual depending on such things as the severity and chronicity of the problem. In short, the longer you've struggled with suicidality, the longer treatment is likely to be. You have the right to withdraw from treatment at any time and if you are dissatisfied with the nature of progress in treatment, an alternative referral will be provided.

CONFIDENTIALITY

The information you convey is confidential and will not be disclosed without your written consent with the exception of the following:

- If you are evaluated to be a danger to yourself or others.
- If your psychologist or provider was appointed by the court to evaluate you.
- If you are a minor, elderly, or disabled and it is believed that you are the victim of abuse, or if you divulge information about abuse.
- If you file suit against the psychologist or provider for breech of duty.
- If a court order or other legal proceedings or statute requires the disclosure of information.
- If you waive the right of privilege or give written consent to disclosure information.
- Anonymous disclosures for audits, evaluations, or research without personally identifying information.
- To third party payers (i.e., those involved in collecting fees for services such as your insurance company).
- Disclosures to other professionals or supervisees directly involved in your treatment or diagnosis.

RECORDS

Documentation of patient visits is kept permanently at the clinic. This generally consists of a summary of each meeting with the psychologist or mental health professional, including diagnosis, clinical markers, treatment provided, recommendations made, and progress (or decline) evidenced.

FEES

Fees are set and collected by the clinic in accordance with institutional policy. It is important for you to meet with someone from the business office in order to review your coverage and decide on a payment plan. It is your responsibility to clarify questions about fees or collection policies with someone from the business office. Questions regarding your insurance carrier should be directed to the business office or your specific carrier. Policies and available benefits vary greatly. We'll work with you to provide any information your insurance carrier needs or establish a payment plan.

If possible, appointments should be cancelled at least 24 hours in advance. If this is done, you will not be charged for missed appointments. Otherwise, a nominal fee will be charged.

EMERGENCY AVAILABILITY

Routine office hours are from 8:00 A.M. to 5:00 P.M., during which time emergency services are available in the clinic. After hours, emergency services are available 24 hours a day through the emergency room and the rotating psychiatrist on call.

QUALIFICATIONS OF YOUR PROVIDER

Information regarding education, training, degrees, and licensure of your provider needs to be directed to him or her.

FIGURE 5.5. *(cont.)*

talization tends to undermine the essential ingredient for any positive therapeutic outcomes—a strong and positive therapeutic alliance (Horvath &
Greenberg, 1994). Given these considerations, it is clearly in the patient's best
interest to provide complete and appropriate informed consent prior to treatment and to carefully structure the therapeutic relationship early on in the
course of developing a viable treatment plan.

If a potentially suicidal patient has received thorough informed consent
about the legal parameters of confidentiality and the importance of outpatient
physical safety, he or she can then proceed in good faith with the clinician toward developing an appropriate treatment plan. As discussed earlier, this kind
of informed consent can be provided to the prospective patient in written form
as well as verbally in the *extended evaluation*. Given this approach, the value
of carefully discussing various aspects of future treatment, as well as the structure of the clinical relationship, cannot be overemphasized. In the spirit of
American Psychological Association ethical guidelines, this might involve extensive detailed discussions of various treatment options and goals, the potential duration of such treatments, fees for service and longer-term costs of treatment (including the limits of managed health care coverage), and various
confidentiality and safety issues. Moreover, clinicians can further clarify their
position on outpatient safety, their availability between sessions, the treatment
techniques they would anticipate using, and other considerations relevant to
the clinical relationship. Patients therefore receive critical front-end information about the potential benefits, costs, time commitment, and other parameters of the available treatment options directly from the clinician so that they
can make their most informed and best choice about their own clinical care
(Rice & Jobes, 1997).

In short, informed consent should include the following: (1) a statement
about the purpose and nature of the services provided, (2) specific therapeutic
goals and procedures to be followed, (3) alternate choices, (4) any identifiable
risks/benefits, (5) the potential duration of treatment, (6) costs and method(s)
of payment, (7) procedures regarding cancellation of appointment(s), (8) constraints on confidentiality, (9) qualifications of the clinician, (10) boundaries
of the professional relationship, and (11) complaint procedures. As evidenced
earlier, use of the conceptual model provides a means to cover all the treatment-related components of informed consent. To cover the others, the clinician can simply add a few paragraphs to the treatment rationale handout detailed in Figure 5.5.

Initiating Self-Monitoring

The final goal is to initiate self-monitoring. Self-monitoring is accomplished
by use of the STR, described earlier in Chapter 2. Figure 5.6 provides a
blank STR and Figure 5.7 a completed STR for Ms. D. The advantages of

the STR are many, including (1) improving the patient's overall emotional awareness, (2) improving the patient's insight and understanding of his or her suicidality, (3) identifying individual-specific treatment targets and scenarios, (4) improving distress tolerance and reducing impulsivity as a simple function of the time invested to complete the STR, (5) improved emotion regulation as a function of providing an organized and structured emotional outlet, (6) an improved sense of emotional control (and related sense of efficacy), (7) serving as a concrete marker of the patient's investment in treatment, and (8) improved communication between clinician and therapist during the treatment process.

In addition to these advantages, it is important to complete any needed consultation, particularly for psychological testing and medication if indicated. The role of psychological testing is discussed later in much more detail. If the steps just summarized are completed, a solid foundation for ongoing treatment will be established, providing the patient with a fairly basic framework within which to understand the problem and, accordingly, invest in the treatment process. For the initial interview, the goal is simply to establish adequate rapport to facilitate ongoing treatment. We have always been impressed by the degree to which a clear and concise rationale for treatment accomplishes this task. The comments made by Ms. D are fairly typical. The final category covered in Table 5.1, the therapeutic relationship, is discussed in detail in the following chapter.

The Use and Role of Psychometric Testing

A Few Comments about Assessment

The psychometric assessment of suicidality can essentially be viewed as an adjunct to the clinical interview. Although there are no data to support any marked predictive validity of existing scales, such scales offer a number of advantages:

- An additional and potentially more objective data source.
- Clarification of different aspects or *factors* of suicidality (e.g., specificity of ideation, plan, intent).
- A potentially less threatening mechanism for the patient to express current thoughts and feelings.
- Introduction of reliability (i.e., consistency) to the assessment process.
- A means to measure potentially subtle changes in suicidality over time and during the course of treatment (and possibly after a particular intervention).

Triggering event(s)[A]	Suicidal thoughts[B]	Severity[C] (1–10)	Duration[D] (1–10)	Feelings[E]	Severity (1–10)	Duration (1–10)	Behavioral response[F]	Charge[G] +/-

[A]Provide as much detail as possible. Indicate the full context, what day, time, who was present, what happened, and what did you do?
[B]Describe the specific thought(s) you had at the time. For example, "I thought of taking an overdose, that I didn't deserve to live, everybody would be better off if I was dead."
[C]Describe the intensity or severity of your thoughts on a scale of 1–10, with 1 being mild and 10 overwhelming.
[D]Note how long the thoughts lasted, a few seconds, minutes, hours, or days. Please try to be precise.
[E]Describe your feelings such as anger, sadness, guilt, anxiety. Remember, you can feel more than one thing at a time.
[F]Describe what you did in response to the trigger and your suicidal thoughts. Remember, doing nothing is doing something!
[G]Please indicate any change in your thoughts or how you felt as a result of your behavioral response, just note it as positive (+) or negative (–).

FIGURE 5.6. Suicidal Thought Record/self-monitoring sheet. From *Treating Suicidal Behavior: An Effective, Time-Limited Approach* by M. David Rudd, Thomas Joiner, and M. Hasan Rajab. Copyright 2001 by The Guilford Press. Permission to reproduce this figure is granted to purchasers of this book for personal use only (see copyright page for details).

Triggering event(s)[A]	Suicidal thoughts[B]	Severity[C] (1–10)	Duration[D] (1–10)	Feelings[E]	Severity (1–10)	Duration (1–10)	Behavioral response[F]	Change[G] +/−
Friday, July 10, 1998, 10:35 P.M. Had an argument with my ex on the phone.	I thought about shooting myself again. Why make an effort?	9	2 minutes.	Anger, frustration, guilt, shame.	9	About 15 minutes.	I went for a walk around the block a couple of times.	++

[A]Provide as much detail as possible. Indicate the full context, what day, time, who was present, what happened, and what did you do?
[B]Describe the specific thought(s) you had at the time. For example, "I thought of taking an overdose, that I didn't deserve to live, everybody would be better off if I was dead."
[C]Describe the intensity or severity of your thoughts on a scale of 1–10, with 1 being mild and 10 overwhelming.
[D]Note how long the thoughts lasted, a few seconds, minutes, hours, or days. Please try to be precise.
[E]Describe your feelings such as anger, sadness, guilt, anxiety. Remember, you can feel more than one thing at a time.
[F]Describe what you did in response to the trigger and your suicidal thoughts. Remember, doing nothing is doing something!
[G]Please indicate any change in your thoughts or how you felt as a result of your behavioral response, just note it as positive (+) or negative (−).

FIGURE 5.7. Example of a completed Suicidal Thought Record/self-monitoring sheet.

The use of assessment instruments helps *balance* the clinician's judgment. Joiner, Rudd, and Rajab (1998a) found that discrepancies occurred between patient self-report and clinician judgment because clinicians took a *better-safe-than-sorry approach*, viewing patients as more suicidal than patients viewed themselves. Interestingly, patients' self-report was better than clinicians' views at predicting suicidality several months later, suggesting that patient self-report has considerable probative value, even when compared to clinician ratings.

The application of psychometric assessment to suicidality takes, for the most part, two forms, incorporating traditional personality testing or measures specific to suicidality. Others have reviewed in detail the role of personality assessment, both objective and projective, in assessing suicidality. Eyman and Eyman (1992) concluded:

- Psychological testing is an important tool for obtaining information crucial to understanding suicidal individuals.
- Suicide screening scales can help identify those potentially at risk among a large group of people.
- Once a person has been identified as at risk, a thorough battery of psychological tests can answer questions about the patient's personality makeup, characteristics that contribute to suicidality, and the circumstances that might lead to suicidal behavior. (p. 141)

We would agree with the recommendations summarized previously, noting that existing personality testing (e.g., MMPI-2 and MCMI-III) can provide a more detailed understanding of personality structure and organization that will ultimately lead to a more refined conceptual model, particularly with respect to predisposing vulnerabilities.

In terms of assessment instruments specific to suicidality, Range and Knott (1997) recently provided a detailed review of the 20 most frequently used and most widely known instruments. They included clinician-rated instruments, self-report suicide instruments, self-report *buffers against suicide* instruments, those focused on children and adolescents, and special-purpose scales. They recommended three scales for use: the Beck Scale for Suicide Ideation (Beck & Steer, 1993), along with its derivative scales (e.g., Modified Scale for Suicide Ideation; Miller et al., 1986); the Reasons for Living Inventory (Linehan, Goodstein, Nielsen, & Chiles, 1983); and the Suicide Behavior Questionnaire (Linehan, 1981).

A Few Practical Considerations

We have found both the Beck Scale for Suicide Ideation (BSS) and the Modified Scale for Suicide Ideation (MSSI) to be very useful. For treatment monitoring purposes, simple and straightforward questions (with careful documentation and ongoing monitoring) such as those summarized in Chapter 6 are most valuable, with periodic integration of formal assessment scales for the reasons summarized previously. We have found that repetitive and frequent use (e.g., weekly) of the scales are often met with considerable resistance and, at times, considerable dissatisfaction and occasionally outright refusal. Infrequent and strategic use (e.g., every 3 months) is accepted by patients without any particular problems. In this fashion, the scales are used to complement clinical judgment and provide a more objective marker of treatment progress (or decline) over time.

Consistent with the recommendation of the American Psychological Association (1998) about psychological assessment in general, the assessment of suicidality relies on a "variety of test-derived pieces of information, obtained from multiple methods of assessment, and placing the data in the context of historical information, referral information, and behavioral observations made during the testing an interview process, in order to generate a cohesive and comprehensive understanding of the person being evaluated" (pp. 107–108). In summary, the clinician should attempt to get as much information as possible; do so in a parsimonious, strategic, and organized fashion; use multiple sources; and repeat the process in a predictable and scheduled manner. In this respect, the initial interview will set the stage for every session to follow.

Establishing the Therapeutic Relationship

Five relatively simple and straightforward steps can be taken to help establish a solid therapeutic relationship and alliance. From the very beginning, in the course of discussing the conceptual model and treatment plan (i.e., informed consent), several specific steps can be taken that target the therapeutic relationship. Included are defining a conceptual framework (Step 1), exploring particular interpersonal problem areas (Steps 2 and 3), defining the necessary language and integrating relationship issues into the treatment agenda (Step 4), and repeating and reviewing over time (Step 5).

Step 1

Conceptualize the therapeutic relationship and alliance as *part* of the treatment agenda; that is, discuss them as a part of the conceptual model offered. The active suicidal mode does not occur in a vacuum. An active suicidal mode, as well as facilitating modes, will affect the very nature of how the patient relates to you and, accordingly, the therapeutic relationship. It is important that they be acknowledged as crucial from the outset. For example:

"If you look back at the conceptual model we discussed, you'll remember that one of the things that consistently triggered your suicidal episodes was interpersonal conflict. Actually, if you want to be
more specific, we could say they happened when you felt rejected in
some way, shape, or form. You mentioned a number of things that
others have done that push this button. I think you said that if someone you feel is important in your life cuts you off in conversation,
doesn't return a phone call, acts disinterested or somehow doesn't
listen, or decides that they don't want to do something with you, all
these trigger feelings of rejection. It's important for us to be able to
discuss these things in therapy because, although it's a therapeutic
relationship, it's still a relationship and from time to time (and probably with greater frequency than I'd like), I'll do some of these things
that will trigger feelings of rejection. As a result, you might get
quite upset and angry, and it might be difficult to talk about, but it is
critically important that we do. Sometimes I may be completely unaware that you're upset, that is, unless you tell me."

Step 2

The clinician should provide historical and developmental context for the current relationship. The most effective way to do this is to draw parallels between developmental history, recurrent interpersonal problems, and how these
patterns might emerge in the therapeutic relationship. For the most part, the
clinician is identifying specific skill deficits that need to be targeted. This
helps the therapeutic relationship by making it clear that these problems are a
part of the treatment agenda and are critical for treatment success. Given that
interpersonal skill deficits affect every relationship the patient has, they will
affect the therapeutic relationship in some manner. Actually, the therapeutic
relationship itself may well be the most effective *vehicle of change*. This is an
area that is often taboo for the patient to talk about and an area that some therapists feel uncomfortable discussing. By emphasizing it, the clinician will
make it *acceptable and expected* that the patient voice these problems and actively discuss them in treatment. Not only will it be acceptable to talk about
relationship problems in treatment, but it will be encouraged and reinforced.
For example:

"We discussed a number of relationship problems that you have had
over the years, and I don't believe it would be inaccurate to say that
those problems have been repeated across different relationships,
even in therapy. Let me give you an example. You said that you always felt criticized and rejected by your mother, and that ever since

that time the problem surfaces in close, intimate relationships. If I re-call it accurately, you stated that when you worry about rejection or abandonment, you either get really angry and 'push people away' or you withdraw and hide, both to 'protect yourself.' So, if we had to translate this to some interpersonal skills to work on, we might say it would be good to work on your ability to tolerate and maintain inti-macy, improve your anger management ability, and develop better trust in relationships. It is very likely, and actually I'd be surprised if some of these problems didn't surface during therapy. Although ther-apy is, in many ways, a unique relationship it is one in which you ad-dress very intimate and potentially threatening material. As a result, it is likely that some of the feelings we just talked about would sur-face in our relationship as well. I just want to make sure that you know it's not only OK to talk about these problems, I believe it es-sential in order to effectively address some of the problems that orig-inally brought you in for treatment."

Step 3

The clinician should ask specific questions about problems the patient has had in previous treatment(s). It is important to know exactly what kinds of inter-personal problems the patient has experienced in previous treatment efforts. Clinicians need to know what to look for and what areas might be particularly hypersensitive. Thus they might be able to anticipate problems. The patient can provide concrete examples that will facilitate discussion of the therapeutic relationship and, simultaneously, facilitate the current relationship. This will also give clinicians some gauge for the patient's degree of insight and under-standing of relationship dynamics. For example:

"Given some of the problems we've discussed about close relation-ships, I was wondering if you ran into any of these problems with your previous therapist(s)? How did you handle them? What made it easier for you to deal with it (them)? What made it more difficult? Did you just stop going? What kind of an impact did this have on you? Did you start feeling hopeless about whether or not treatment can help?"

Step 4

The clinician should provide the patient a specific framework and language for discussing the therapeutic relationship. Specifically, the clinician should set the boundaries for targeting this problem. This is routinely an overwhelming issue for many suicidal patients. If the clinician does not provide a framework and language for them, it is highly unlikely that they will understand how to broach the subject. For example:

> "When the therapy relationship comes up, you might want to think about a few specific things. If you don't mind, I would encourage you to think about your feeling about treatment in general, that is, whether or not you think things are going well, what's working and what's not. You also might want to consider how you see my role, whether or not I'm doing a good job, if you feel I've got things on the right track, If I'm focused, giving you enough time, promptly returning calls, among many other possible things. Also, are we in agreement about the problems and how to resolve them? The last thing I'd encourage you to consider is how you're feeling about your own role in treatment, that is, what things are you responsible for, what things you're doing well, what things you're struggling with, as well as whether or not you feel capable of working on and making the kind of changes we're talking about."

Step 5

The clinician should make repetition and review routine and consistent items on the treatment agenda (e.g., he or she should designate a few minutes at the end of every third or fourth session to address the therapeutic relationship specifically). Repetition and review are critical. As is clear from the treatment model discussed so far, the therapeutic relationship is essential to success but it does not need to become the only focus of treatment. They are critical items on the treatment agenda, but as reviewed previously, there are many others. There are other concrete targets and considerable time needs to be devoted to them. It is important to place the therapeutic relationship in proper perspective. Otherwise, as is discussed in detail later, manipulation and misuse of the relationship can become central problems. For example:

> "I'm glad we've had the opportunity to discuss the therapy relationship in more detail. It's my thought that this needs to be done on a periodic basis, maybe every couple of weeks or once a month, or whenever the circumstances demand it. It's important that you feel comfortable enough to bring up your concerns. I know this won't be easy, especially early on in treatment. Please let me know if there's anything I can do to make this process easier for you. What are your thoughts and feelings about what I've said so far?"

Clearly, the therapeutic relationship needs to be addressed in a consistent manner throughout the course of treatment. Many challenges, however, face the clinician working with the acutely or chronically suicidal patient. At times, it will feel as if the patient simply does not want therapy to work. It is perhaps more accurate to say that some suicidal patients will simply *not know how to make therapy work*. Dealing effectively with disruptions and provocations in treatment will help patients learn the skills necessary and make the changes needed for lasting recovery.

6

Assessing Suicide Risk

The assessment of suicidal thinking and related behaviors is an area of critical importance for all practicing clinicians, with errors of omission or commission carrying disproportionate risk for a tragic outcome. Treating suicidal behavior on an outpatient basis demands a systematic approach to risk assessment and related day-to-day management. This is particularly true when access to care is restricted or seriously limited in terms of frequency, type, or duration.

Recently, specific practice guidelines in suicidality have been offered addressing risk assessment, treatment, and emergency management (Rudd, Joiner, Jobes, & King, 1999). These guidelines, although limited in scope, are based on available empirical research rather than identified *failure scenarios* in clinical practice. Previous guidelines have been rooted in clinical failure scenarios, or retrospective judgments of *what was done wrong* rather than what we know works from a scientific standpoint. Nonetheless, they still represent the published standard of care to which practicing clinicians will be held, or at least evaluated against, when there is an unfortunate clinical outcome (Bongar et al., 1992; Bongar et al., 1993; Silverman et al., 1994).

This chapter provides a general framework for the ongoing assessment of suicidality in outpatient practice. It is compatible with both the existing standards of care and more recent recommended practice guidelines. The framework provided is consistent with the CBT model presented earlier (i.e., the suicidal mode) and is based on applicable empirical research. It is estimated that up to one-third of the general population acknowledges suicidal ideation at some point during their lives and far greater numbers of those presenting in a psychiatric setting note at least some suicidality (Paykel,

Myers, Lindenthal, & Tanner, 1974; Schwab, Warheit, & Holzer, 1972). A surprising number of clinicians, nonetheless, fail to use a consistent or comprehensive assessment model in inpatient and outpatient settings alike (Jobes, Eyman, & Yufit, 1990).

In addition to providing a risk assessment framework for outpatient practice and related clinical decision making, this chapter also addresses the following topics, all of which are critical to both a thorough understanding of risk assessment and competent clinical practice in the area of suicidality:

1. Differentiating between the tasks of risk assessment and prediction.
2. The importance of precision and consistency in our use of terminology.
3. The often neglected but critical role of *time* in risk assessment.
4. The need to engage in *risk monitoring* by establishing a category of both risk and related severity.
5. The importance of thorough and complete documentation.
6. Assessing risk in chronically suicidal patients.
7. The implications for ongoing management and treatment, particularly in time-limited settings.

Distinguishing between Risk Assessment and Prediction: Defining the Nature of Clinical Responsibilities

An expectation exists in the legal community and the court system that a clinician can predict his or her patient's suicidal or homicidal behavior: the legal concept is foreseeability. Without question, such an expectation is problematic for the practicing clinician for several reasons. First, it makes an unrealistic clinical demand on the therapist. As a result, it raises the anxiety of the clinician, potentially influencing the very nature of day-to-day practice and related clinical procedures. For example, much more time than necessary may be spent conducting risk assessment evaluations, doing psychometric testing, or requesting professional consultations, as a means of overcompensating for this anxiety, rather than providing psychotherapeutic treatment. Also, the court-generated expectation that clinicians can reliably predict their patients' behavior actually influences the existing standard of care with this population, regardless of available empirical findings. The idea of suicide prediction has persisted both in the court system and clinical office despite considerable evidence that the expectation is simply unrealistic.

Low base-rate phenomena such as suicide are impossible to predict with any reliability in an individual case, simply by nature of the statistical problem presented. Actually, we would be correct more often than not simply to predict that a patient *would not* commit suicide, regardless of the clinical presentation.

Empirical suicide prediction models have consistently demonstrated this point, resulting in inordinately high false-positive and false-negative rates and proving to have little, if any, practical utility (e.g., Clark, Young, Scheftner, Fawcett, & Fogg, 1987; Mackinnon & Farberow, 1975; Motto, Heilbron, & Juster, 1985; Murphy, 1972, 1983, 1984; Pokorny, 1983, 1992).

The available research in this area is relatively straightforward. We are not in the business of predicting suicide, simply assessing risk in a reasonable, reliable, consistent, and clinically useful manner. It is important for the practicing clinician to use an assessment model that communicates this idea and to document accordingly. Such a model balances both risk and protective factors, emphasizes the inherent fallacy of prediction, and provides a straightforward presentation of empirically grounded risk variables. Ideally, the model employed for risk assessment would be conceptually consistent with the theoretical approach to treatment. If so, risk assessment becomes a natural, meaningful, and vital part of the treatment process itself, one essential to good care and something difficult to casually dismiss.

The fact that we cannot reliably predict suicidal behavior does not mean we have not identified salient risk factors that place a patient in what Litman (1990) has referred to as the suicide zone. The clinician's task is to recognize when the patient has entered this risk zone (i.e., risk assessment) and to respond accordingly (i.e., management and treatment). Risk assessment can both *explain and estimate* the patient's suicidality. It is indistinguishable from the treatment process, not a separate task or demand. It is essentially a *treatment map* that answers questions critical to the patient's immediate and ongoing care, questions consistent with the underlying CBT theory presented earlier.

The Importance of Precise Terminology: Saying What We Know and Knowing What We Say

An essential first step in accurate risk assessment is the use of a standard nomenclature. Without a standard nomenclature, the clinician gambles that assessments and communication with the patient will be misinterpreted simply as a function of inconsistent or imprecise terminology. In other words, we may *mean* to say one thing but inadvertently convey another and vice versa for our patients. In a managed care environment, if we meant to denote high risk but imply that the behavior is chronic and essentially the function of personality disturbance (e.g., borderline *acting out or repeated gestures*), the high-risk nature of the case may not be clearly communicated. As a result, treatment may well be restricted and the opportunity for follow-up care lost until the next *gesture*.

O'Carroll et al. (1996) recently proposed a standard nomenclature, offering descriptive terminology that falls into two broad categories: instrumental behavior (i.e., zero intent to die with other motivation such as help-seeking, punishing others, or attention-seeking) and suicidal acts (i.e., intent to die). Figure 6.1 provides a detailed listing of the nomenclature offered, specifying the differences across each with respect to intent and outcome. Those definitions that will most frequently be employed in day-to-day clinical practice include the following:

> *Suicide:* Death from injury, poisoning, or suffocation where there is evidence (either implicit or explicit) that the injury was self-inflicted and that the decedent intended to kill himself/herself. Note: the term completed suicide can be used interchangeably with the term suicide.
>
> *Suicide attempt with injuries:* An action resulting in nonfatal injury, poisoning, or suffocation where there is evidence (either implicit or explicit) that the injury was self-inflicted and that he/she intended at some level to kill himself/herself.
>
> *Suicide attempt without injuries:* A potentially self-injurious behavior with a nonfatal outcome, for which there is evidence (either implicit or explicit) that the person intended at some level to kill himself/herself.
>
> *Instrumental suicide-related behavior:* Potentially self-injurious behavior for which there is evidence (either implicit or explicit) that the person did not intend to kill himself/herself (i.e., zero intent to die) and the person wished to use the appearance of intending to kill himself/herself in order to attain some other end (e.g., to seek help, to punish others, or to receive attention). Instrumental suicide-related behavior can occur with injuries, without injuries, or with fatal outcome (i.e., accidental death).
>
> *Suicide threat:* Any interpersonal action, verbal or nonverbal, stopping short of a directly self-harmful act, that a reasonable person would interpret as communicating or suggesting that a suicidal act or other suicide-related behavior might occur in the near future.
>
> *Suicidal ideation:* Any self-reported thoughts of engaging in suicide-related behavior. (pp. 246 247)

As discussed previously, the use of a standard nomenclature has a number of identifiable advantages for the practicing clinician. Perhaps most important, though, is that the terminology offered is descriptive and observational in nature. The proposed nomenclature distinguishes three essential elements of suicide-related behavior (e.g., Maris et al., 1992): (1) outcome (i.e., injury, no injury, or death), (2) evidence of self-infliction, and (3) evidence of intent to die by suicide (i.e., both implicit and explicit intent). The recognition of the importance of these elements and their integration into the terminology provides the practicing clinician an opportunity to more clearly document the critical role played by intent. In particular, it serves to acknowledge the variable nature of intent over time, the difficulty of accurately assessing intent under certain conditions (e.g., a purposefully misleading and treat-

Terms for suicide-related behaviors			Intent to die from suicide*	Instrumental thinking	Outcome		
					No injury	Nonfatal injury	Death
Suicide-related behavior	Instrumental Behavior	Instrumental suicide related behavior					
		—With injuries	No	Yes		★	
		—Without injuries	No	Yes	★		
		Fatal outcome †	No	Yes			★
	Suicidal acts	Suicide attempt					
		—With injuries	Yes	+/−		★	
		—Without injuries	Yes	+/−	★		
		Completed suicide	Yes	+/−			★

FIGURE 6.1. Proposed standard nomenclature. *Conscious intent to end one's life through the suicidal behavior; †considered accidental death.

ment resistant patient), and the resultant dilemma and fallacy of reliably predicting a patient's behavior.

Intent is a subjective, personal motivation, one communicated in both implicit and explicit ways. Certainly, patients can tell us what their intent is if we ask during the interview (i.e., explicit or subjective intent). There are, however, other means of assessing intent (i.e., implicit or objective intent) based on behavioral markers. Beck and Lester (1976) originally provided objective and subjective markers of intent, consistent with the conceptualization and nomenclature provided by O'Carroll et al. (1996). Objective markers include characteristics such as timing of the attempt, isolation, precautions taken against discovery, acting to get help, final acts in preparation of death, leaving a suicide note, lethality of method, degree of premeditation and planning, and prior suicide attempts (Beck & Lester, 1976). Subjective markers include not only the expressed purpose of the behavior (i.e., stated intent) but also prior communications, expectations of fatality and expressed understanding of the lethality of the behavior, attitude toward dying, beliefs about the probability for rescue, and reaction to surviving the attempt. These markers are integrated into the assessment framework provided later in the chapter.

Essential Components of a Clinical Risk Assessment Interview

This section focuses specifically on the clinical interview exploring suicidality. Chapter 5 addresses the use of psychometric assessment instruments in coordinated fashion. Here we present a method for restructuring the assessment interview, distinguish between the four identified categories of risk, and elaborate on the questions to ask in order to rate the severity of risk. In addition, we offer a continuum of suicidality for rating severity within each of the four risk categories.

Naturally, the assessment of suicidality is only one component of the clinical interview and assessment process and should not be considered in isolation. The assumption here is that a complete intake history and diagnostic interview have also been completed, psychological testing used and integrated when possible, and interviews with significant others conducted when available. Each of these is discussed in much more detail in Chapter 5.

The categories for risk assessment include the following: predisposition to suicidal behavior, identifiable precipitant or stressors, the patient's symptomatic presentation, the presence of hopelessness, the nature of the patient's suicidal thinking, previous suicidal behavior, impulsivity and self-control, and identifiable protective factors.

Figure 6.2 provides a detailed listing of the variables covered within each domain, a principal organizational question that needs to be answered, and specific questions for each component. Consistent with others (e.g., Clark & Fawcett, 1992; Rudd & Joiner, 1998; Somers-Flanagan & Somers-Flanagan, 1995), we recommend a specific sequence to questioning, moving from the identifiable precipitant to the patient's symptomatic presentation to hopelessness and ultimately to the nature of the patient's suicidal thinking. In so moving, the suicidal mode and the corresponding belief system are both defined.

The sequenced approach recommended has several advantages. Perhaps most important is the possible reduction in anxiety and agitation and improved rapport as the result of a gradual progression in the intensity and therapeutic intimacy of the interview. At two different transition points in the interview, the clinician is provided with a unique opportunity to normalize the patient's manifest anxiety, improve rapport, and ensure a more accurate risk assessment. For example, as the interview progresses and the clinician transitions from a discussion of the patient's presenting symptoms to the possible emergence of hopelessness, he or she can simply add, "It's not unusual for someone that is depressed and experiencing significant stress to feel hopeless. Have you felt hopeless lately?" This one statement normalizes the patient's manifest psychopathology within the context of the presenting disorder (e.g., a major depressive episode) and, as a result, reduces anxiety, resistance, and improves rapport. The net result is likely to be a more honest report on the part of the

Category I: Predisposition to suicidal behavior (predisposing vulnerabilities)

Does the patient have a predisposition to suicidal behavior? This question is routinely answered during the context of an intake interview and history.
Consider the following:

A. Previous history of psychiatric diagnoses (increased risk with recurrent disorders, comorbidity, and chronicity).
B. Previous history of suicidal behavior (increased risk with previous attempts, high lethality, and chronic disturbance).
A specific questioning sequence is offered below.
C. History of abuse (i.e., physical, sexual, emotional), family violence, or punitive parenting: "Can you tell me about your family, what your childhood and adolescent years were like? Were you ever the victim of abuse—physical, sexual, or emotional— either by your parents, a family member, or anyone else. Can you tell me more about it? Was there violence of any type in your family? Can you tell me more about it? How did your parents discipline you (and your siblings)?"

Category II: Precipitants or stressors (triggers)

What triggered the suicidal crisis?
Consider the following:

A. Review any significant loss—financial, interpersonal relationship(s), identity: "How have things been going for you recently? At home? At work? In your relationship with . . . [significant others]? Can you tell me about anything in particular that has been stressful for you?"
B. Address any acute or chronic health problems: "Tell me about your health? Have you had any problems recently?" If chronic pain is an issue: "Have you had difficulty managing your pain recently? What are you doing to manage your pain?"
C. Address any possible family instability: "How are things at home? Tell me about your relationship with . . . your spouse . . . children . . . parents . . . partner?"

Category III: Symptomatic presentation (affective system)

What kind of symptom picture does the patient present?
Consider the following:

A. Axis I and II diagnoses, with a particular focus on depression and anxiety: "Have you been feeling sad, depressed, down, or blue lately? Which of the following have you experienced: difficulty sleeping . . . poor energy . . . either poor or increased appetite (with weight loss or gain) . . . a lack of interest in things . . . negative feelings about yourself . . . difficulty concentrating or focusing . . . guilt feelings . . . thoughts about death or dying? Have you been feeling anxious, nervous, or panicky lately?"
B. Severity of symptoms: "How bad has your depression been? Can you rate it on a sale of 1 to 10 . . . with 1 being the best you've ever felt and 10 being so depressed that you couldn't function or you've seriously contemplated suicide? How bad has your anxiety been? Can you rate it on a scale of 1 to 10 . . . with 1 being no anxiety at all and completely calm and 10 being so anxious and tense that you couldn't sit still and would do anything for relief? What have you been doing to get relief from the anxiety?"

(continued)

FIGURE 6.2. Risk assessment categories and hierarchical questioning. From Rudd and Joiner (1998b). Copyright 1998 by Professional Resource Exchange. Reprinted by permission.

C. Presence of anger, agitation, and/or a sense of urgency: "Have you felt angry or agitated lately? If so, can you rate its severity on a scale of 1 to 10 . . . with 1 being no anger and 10 being so angry or agitated you thought you were going to lose control? Have you felt a sense of urgency lately, like you needed to do something quickly for relief? If so, what have you done to get relief . . . drink . . . use drugs . . . use prescription medications . . . something to harm yourself in any way?"

D. Comorbidity: Questions to address the co-occurrence of any of the above. For example, "Have you been feeling depressed, anxious , angry, or agitated at the same time?"

Category IV: Presence of hopelessness
(cognitive system, suicidal belief system)

Is the patient hopeless?
Consider the following:

A. Presence of hopelessness: "Have you felt hopeless lately . . . like things wouldn't improve or get better?"

B. Severity of hopelessness: "Could you rate the severity of your hopelessness on a scale of 1 to 10 . . . 1 being optimistic about the future and 10 being utterly hopeless about things getting better for you?"

Category V: The nature of suicidal thinking
(cognitive system, suicidal belief system)

What is the nature of the patient's current suicidal thinking?
Consider the following:

A. Current ideation frequency, intensity, and duration: "Do you ever have thoughts of killing yourself . . . thoughts of suicide? If so, can you tell me exactly what you think about? How often do you think about killing yourself . . . daily . . . weekly . . . monthly? How many times a day? How long do the thoughts usually last . . . a few seconds . . . a few minutes . . . hours . . . longer? How severe, intense, or overwhelming are the thoughts? Could you rate the severity or intensity on a scale of 1to 10, with 1 being mild and 10 being severe and overwhelming?"

B. Specificity and plans: "Can you tell me specifically what you've been thinking . . . how you would kill yourself? When people think about suicide, they often think about how, when, and where . . . have you had these kinds of thoughts? Have you thought of any other method of suicide? Do you have a plan for how you would kill yourself with [method]?"

C. Availability of means: "Do you have [method] available to you or do you have access to [method]? If so, where? If not, have you made arrangements to get [method]?"

D. Active behaviors: "Have you acted on these thoughts in any way? Have you taken any steps in preparation for killing yourself? If so, what steps have you taken . . . what have you done?"

E. Explicit (i.e., subjective) intent: "Do you have any intention of acting on the thoughts of suicide? Could you rate your intent on a scale of 1 to 10, with 1 being no intention of acting on the thoughts and 10 being certain that you'll act on them the first chance you get? Have you talked with anyone about your suicidal thoughts? What are your beliefs about death/dying? What do you think will happen? How did you feel about surviving your last attempt (i.e., if a previous attempt)?"

F. Deterrents to suicide: "You haven't acted on these thoughts yet . . . what keeps you alive right now . . . what keeps you going? What's kept you going in the past when you've had these thoughts?"

(continued)

FIGURE 6.2. *(cont.)*

Category VI: Previous suicidal behavior, preparatory behaviors (behavioral system)

Does the patient have a previous history of suicidal behavior? Has the patient engaged in any identifiable preparatory behaviors?
Consider the following:

A. Frequency and context: How many suicide attempts have you made in your lifetime? Starting with the first one, can you tell me about what was going on at the time . . . what precipitated it?"
B. Perceived lethality and outcome (i.e., helps assess implicit or objective intent) of each attempt: "Did you think [method] would kill you? Did you receive medical care? If so, what kind? Did you receive psychiatric care? If so, what kind and for how long? How did you feel about surviving?"
C. Opportunity for rescue and help-seeking (i.e., helps assess implicit or objective intent): "How did you get help after the suicide attempt? Who discovered you? What were the circumstances? Do you take any steps to ensure that you wouldn't be discovered? If so, what?"
D. Preparatory behaviors of any type: "What preparatory behaviors, planning, rehearsal behaviors, or attempts has the patient engaged in? Common preparatory behaviors include things like financial planning, writing letters to loved ones, purchasing insurance or making changes in insurance coverage, completing or altering a will, accessing the means to suicide, organizing materials to suicide, or actually rehearsing the suicide.

Category VII: Impulsivity and self-control (behavioral system)

Is the patient impulsive? Does he or she lack self-control?
Consider the following:

A. Subjective self-control: "Do you consider yourself impulsive? If so, why? Do you feel in control right now? If not, why? Have you had times recently when you felt out of control? What were you doing? Could you rate how much in control you feel on a scale of 1 to 10, with 1 being in complete control and 10 completely out of control? Do you feel like you can control your suicidal impulses?"
B. Objective control: "Have you been drinking or using a substance of any type? If so, assess frequency, magnitude of abuse, duration, and presence of substances. Have you had problems with impulsive behavior of any type . . . sexual acting out . . . aggressive acting out?"

Category VIII: Protective factors

What protective factors are present?
Consider the following:

A. Social support—family and friends: "Do you have family or friends available that you can talk to and depend on? Have you accessed them for support? If not, why? Do you have anyone that you can turn to for help in a crisis?"
B. Problem-solving and coping history: "Have you had trouble solving problems and coping in the past? Do you have trouble identifying solutions or seeing answers to your current problems?"
C. Active treatment: "Are you actively in psychotherapy . . . on medications . . . or both? How have you responded to treatment in the past . . . have you found it helpful?"
D. Hopefulness: "Do you have times when you feel hopeful or optimistic about your situation?"

FIGURE 6.2. *(cont.)*

patient and, accordingly, a more accurate risk assessment. Similarly, the clinician can ease the transition from a discussion of hopelessness to suicidal thinking by noting, "It's not uncommon for someone who's been overly stressed, clinically depressed, and hopeless to have thoughts about suicide. Have you?"

Tips on Eliciting Information on Intent and Self-Control

Although Figure 6.2 is, for the most part, self-explanatory, several points deserve special emphasis. As noted in the discussion about terminology, it is important to recognize and distinguish between explicit (i.e., subjective) and implicit (i.e., objective) intent. Distinguishing between the two is consistent with the original conceptualization of suicide intent offered by Beck and Lester (1976). Explicit or subjective intent is simply the patient's stated intent. How do patients respond when the clinician asks them whether they have any intention of acting on their thoughts? What is their attitude about dying? How did they feel about surviving the attempt? What did they think was the probability for rescue? What was their understanding of the lethality of the method chosen? In contrast, objective or implicit intent is further estimated by the patient's current and past behaviors (e.g., timing of the attempt, efforts made to prevent rescue or discovery prior to a suicide attempt, help-seeking behavior after an attempt, extensive prepatory behaviors such as putting financial affairs in order prior to an attempt or leaving a suicide note, and choice of highly lethal method).

Ideally, there would be concordance between statements of intent and objective indicators. It is not uncommon, however, to get conflicting reports. This is often the case with chronically suicidal patients. In these cases, we recommend that the clinician give disproportionate weight to objective markers of intent when assessing risk.

As indicated in Figure 6.2, we have also distinguished between objective and subjective markers of self-control. Similar to the construct of intent, this provides a means of more closely evaluating the accuracy of a patient's self-report. A comment is also warranted about questioning the patient about method(s). We strongly recommend asking at least twice what method(s) the patient has considered. It is as simple as asking, "Have you considered any other methods?" after the patient has discussed the initial one. It is not uncommon for a suicidal patient to withhold the most lethal or accessible method until questioned further. We have encountered this pattern most frequently with chronically suicidal and personality-disordered patients. In many ways, it represents the ambivalence that is the hallmark of the suicidal crisis and a test of the clinician's clinical resolve and commitment, as well as evidence of underlying personality psychopathology.

We have also found it extremely useful to use simple 1-to-10 rating scales when questioning suicidal patients. Such rating scales are perhaps most useful in addressing the severity of presenting symptoms, anger, hopelessness, current suicidal thoughts, explicit intent, and self-control. Although simple procedures, the advantages are numerous. First, rating scales provide a mechanism by which the patient can both quantify and clarify a subjective emotional experience. Second, the ratings allow for comparisons over time and adjustments in risk assessment ratings. Third, such scales provide a simple means by which the patient can both recognize and monitor fluctuations (and most importantly improvement) in symptom-level variables. This is something that patients often have marked difficulty with during periods of acute crisis characterized by hopelessness. The numerical ratings provide a somewhat objective marker that can be shared with the patient in order to emphasize and demonstrate that change and progress do, in fact, occur even though the subjective emotional experience continues to be painful. And, finally, such scales can potentially improve communication between the many clinicians involved in the patient's care, ideally, improving resultant management and treatment. As is frequently the case with suicidal patients, a little bit of structure often goes a long way.

As is evident from the model presented and the questions asked, risk assessment in many ways helps delineate the patient's suicidal belief system and the *content* of the suicidal mode. Conceptualizing the patient's suicidality, assessing risk, and articulating a specific treatment plan are all inextricably intertwined. A lack of specificity and focus in any one area influences the other two and vice versa. Consistent with this line of thinking, risk assessment is a continuous task in the treatment of suicidal patients. In addition to the usual approach of rating risk severity, we also distinguish between four categories of risk: baseline, acute, chronic high risk, and chronic high risk with acute exacerbation. In summary, risk assessment involves two distinct steps: (1) designating the risk category and (2) rating severity.

Risk Categories: Baseline, Acute, Chronic High Risk, and Chronic High Risk with Acute Exacerbation

In accordance with the previous discussion, we recommend that clinicians distinguish between the four risk categories designated in Table 6.1. Baseline risk is that level of risk presented by the patient when not in a state of acute crisis, that is, when symptoms and stressors have resolved. Essentially, baseline risk is present when the patient is asymptomatic, that is, at his or her *relative best*. All suicidal individuals, whether ideators, single attempters, or chronic multiple attempters, have a baseline risk rating that they *return to* during periods of relative calm and remission of psychopathology.

TABLE 6.1. Suicide risk categories.

Risk category	Criteria
I. Baseline	Absence of an acute (i.e., crisis) overlay, no significant stressors nor prominent symptomatology. Only appropriate for ideators and single attempters.
II. Acute	Presence of acute (i.e., crisis) overlay, significant stressor(s) and/or prominent symptomatology. Only appropriate for ideators and single attempters.
III. Chronic high risk	Baseline risk for multiple attempters. Absence of an acute (i.e., crisis) overlay, no significant stressors nor prominent symptomatology.
IV. Chronic high risk with acute exacerbation	Acute risk category for multiple attempters. Presence of acute (i.e., crisis) overlay, significant stressor(s) and/or prominent symptomatology.

Baseline risk is not, however, comparable across each of these groups. The use of simple severity ratings implies comparability, hence, the need for categorization *and* ratings of severity.

Depending on history, all suicidal patients have different levels of severity of baseline risk. A return to baseline risk is the initial treatment target, consistent with the notion of symptom remission. The concept of baseline risk serves a simple and straightforward purpose in treatment planning. It represents a reasonable initial goal for time-limited treatment. In other words, what is the best the patient can expect given his or her current abilities and skill level, symptomatically and functionally? A reduction or significant change of baseline risk would actually necessitate enduring individual change secondary to fundamental personality change (e.g., development, refinement and generalization of problem-solving or coping skills, self-image change, and lasting change in interpersonal copying style). Naturally, this would involve longer-term treatment. One of the primary goals of time-limited treatment is a return to baseline risk, not substantial modification of baseline severity. Baseline risk can and should be established for any psychiatric patient presenting clinically, regardless of whether or not there is an active suicidal component.

In contrast, acute risk is that level of risk presented during an acute suicidal crisis, when the patient is symptomatic and *at his or her worst*. Acute risk is estimated for ideators and single attempters only. By definition, acute risk is time limited. It may only endure for a few minutes, hours, or days. Chronic high risk is a category reserved for those evidencing long-standing suicidal behaviors and making multiple suicide attempts. There is a growing body of evidence to suggest that those making multiple attempts are at greater risk relative to ideators and single attempters and present a more severe clinical picture (e.g., Clark & Fawcett, 1992; Maris, 1992; Rudd, Joiner, & Rajab, 1996).

The category of chronic high risk provides a means of clearly articulating and communicating that the baseline risk level is always elevated in contrast to other patients and that the patient is always considered at high risk. In other words, even at his or her best, the patient still poses substantial risk. It is a straightforward method of denoting the enduring severity of the psycho-pathology presented, across both Axis I and II, regardless of whether an acute crisis has resolved. As with any rating scheme, severity of risk is always rela-tive. Accordingly, the variable nature of suicidality, even among those at chronic high risk, can be acknowledged by adding, when necessary, the descriptor of *acute exacerbation*. For example, when there is an acute stressor or marked reemergence of Axis I symptomatology, the patient can be de-scribed as *chronic high risk with acute exacerbation*. This communicates the time-limited elevation of risk, even for those falling in this high-risk category.

Rating Severity: A Continuum of Suicidality

Somers-Flanagan and Somers-Flanagan (1995) proposed a continuum of suicidality ranging from nonexistent to extreme, based on a number of iden-tifiable risk factors. Their continuum has been modified somewhat, incorpo-rating a more precise conceptualization of intent along with the nomencla-ture proposed by O'Carroll et al. (1996), integrating the role of chronic suicidal behavior, and considering protective factors. Essentially, application of a continuum of suicidality is consistent with an effort to more precisely place the individual patient in what Litman (1990) referred to as the *suicide zone* and to respond accordingly, not to predict the patient's suicidal behav-ior. Our clinical responsibility and obligation are to do a thorough job in our assessment of risk and to respond accordingly, that is, to provide competent clinical management and treatment. To do this we need to know what infor-mation is important, what questions to ask, and how to integrate the infor-mation in a coherent and meaningful framework to guide subsequent clinical decision making.

The following continuum of suicidality is recommended for severity rat-ings:

1. *Nonexistent*: No identifiable suicidal ideation.
2. *Mild*: Suicidal ideation of limited frequency, intensity, and duration, no identifiable plans no intent (i.e., subjective or objective), mild dysphoria/symptomatology, good self-control (i.e., subjective and ob-jective), few risk factors, and identifiable protective factors.

3. *Moderate*: Frequent suicidal ideation with limited intensity and dura-
    tion, some specific plans, no intent (i.e., subjective or objective),
    good self-control (i.e., subjective and objective), limited dysphoria/
    symptomatology, some risk factors present, identifiable protective
    factors.
4. *Severe*: Frequent, intense, and enduring suicidal ideation, specific
    plans, no subjective intent but some objective markers of intent (e.g.,
    choice of lethal method(s), the method is available/accessible, some
    limited prepatory behavior), evidence of impaired self-control (i.e.,
    subjective and/or objective), severe dysphoria/symptomatology, mul-
    tiple risk factors present, few if any protective factors.
5. *Extreme*: Frequent, intense, enduring suicidal ideation, specific
    plans, clear subjective and objective intent, impaired self-control (i.e.,
    subjective and objective), severe dysphoria/symptomatology (i.e.,
    psycheache), many risk factors, no protective factors. As is evident in
    the continuum offered, intent is a critical determinant of risk and, ac-
    cordingly, subsequent clinical decision making.

Each category covered in the clinical interview (i.e., Figure 6.2, sections
I–VIII) can be rated independently, coupled with an overall rating of severity.
Depending on the nature of the clinical presentation (i.e., ideator, single attempter, and multiple attempter), the category of risk can also be designated.
As outlined in Figure 6.3, a *risk monitoring card* can be used from session to
session to supplement clinical entries, summarizing pertinent information in
an easily accessible format. Regardless of the procedures implemented, several points need to be remembered. First, a detailed and structured assessment
system is critical to outpatient practice and accurate risk assessment. Second,
initial and subsequent assessments need to be thoroughly documented; initial
risk categories designated, and associated ratings established. Third, the assessment procedures employed need to recognize the variable and time-
limited nature of acute risk (even for those making multiple attempts) and allow for modifications in risk ratings across sessions. In other words, if the patient falls into either the "acute" or the "chronic high risk with acute exacerbation" categories, it is clear that the patient is in crisis. Subsequent entries will
eventually need to indicate resolution of this acute risk with a return to either
baseline risk or chronic high risk. This addresses previously raised concerns
about the issue of *forseeability* of suicidality. Even for those who have made
numerous attempts, we can never be certain of future episodes. And, finally,
the risk ratings need to translate directly to day-to-day clinical decision making and service provisions. The variables covered in the clinical interview and
outlined in Figure 6.2 provide specific treatment targets, directly tied to fluctuations in severity of risk.

Risk category: 1. Baseline
                     2. Acute
                     3. Chronic high risk
                     4. Chronic high risk with acute exacerbation

Severity ratings:

1. Predisposing vulnerabilities: 1 (Nonexistent) _____ 2 (Mild) _____
   3 (Moderate) _____ 4 (Severe) _____ 5 (Extreme)
   Notes:

2. Precipitant or triggers: 1 (None) _____ 2 (Mild) _____
   3 (Moderate) _____ 4 (Severe) _____ 5 (Extreme)
   Notes:

3. Symptomatic presentation: 1 (None) _____ 2 (Mild) _____
   3 (Moderate) _____ 4 (Severe) _____ 5 (Extreme)
   Notes:

4. Hopelessness: 1 (None) _____ 2 (Mild) _____ 3 (Moderate) _____
   4 (Severe) _____ 5 (Extreme)
   Notes:

5. Suicidal thinking: 1 (None) _____ 2 (Mild) _____ 3 (Moderate) _____
   4 (Severe) _____ 5 (Extreme)
   Notes:

6. Prior suicidal behavior: 1 (None) _____ 2 (Mild) _____
   3 (Moderate) _____ 4 (Severe) _____ 5 (Extreme)
   Notes:

7. Impulsivity and self-control: 1 (None) _____ 2 (Mild) _____
   3 (Moderate) _____ 4 (Severe) _____ 5 (Extreme)
   Notes:

8. Protective factors: 1 (Many) _____ 2 (Substantial) _____
   3 (Moderate) _____ 4 (Few) _____ 5 (None)
   Notes:

Overall rating of risk severity: 1 (Nonexistent) _____ 2 (Mild) _____
3 (Moderate) _____ 4 (Severe) _____ 5 (Extreme)
Summary of significant indicators:

FIGURE 6.3. Risk monitoring card. From *Treating Suicidal Behavior: An Effective, Time-Limited Approach* by M. David Rudd, Thomas Joiner, and M. Hasan Rajab. Copyright 2001 by The Guilford Press. Permission to reproduce this figure is granted to purchasers of this book for personal use only (see copyright page for details).

Clinical Documentation and the Process of Risk: The Concept of Risk Monitoring

The importance of careful documentation in the management and treatment of suicidal patients has been well stated elsewhere, with clear and comprehensive coverage of the necessary content of clinical files (e.g., Bongar, 1992; VandeCreek & Knapp, 1989). Rather than address issues of content, we would like to provide a brief discussion on the importance of considering the *process of risk* over time and how this relates to documentation. Most clinicians would agree that the assessment of suicide risk is not a static process but one that varies over time, in accordance with the severity and intensity of the variables summarized previously. It is not uncommon to have dramatic shifts in risk over periods as brief as a day. The use of simple severity ratings implies comparability, hence, the need for categorization *and* ratings of severity.

As discussed previously, some current work suggests distinct, and clinically important, differences between the three groups of ideators, attempters, and multiple attempters (e.g., Clark & Fawcett, 1992; Maris, 1992; Rudd, Joiner, & Rajab, 1996). In particular, there appear to be distinct differences in baseline risks for multiple attempters, even under the *best of conditions*. In contrast to single attempters or ideators, it may well be that their risk rating is always elevated as a result of the type, chronicity, and severity of psychopathology. This clinical possibility is easily communicated by carefully documenting and designating chronic high risk in contrast to baseline risk for ideators and single attempters.

Initial baseline and recurrent suicide risk assessments will ideally translate into straightforward, clinically indicated, and effective decision making. To do so, both initial and subsequent suicide risk assessment ratings need to be linked directly to specific criteria, with their status subsequently monitored and modified over time in the clinical chart. In addition, clinical decisions and interventions need to target changes in risk, that is, those variables linked to a change in status. Take, for example, the following brief clinical vignette:

Case of Mr. Z

A 25-year-old single white male was referred for psychiatric evaluation following a conflict with his ex-girlfriend. The patient was picked up by the police at his ex-girlfriend's house. At the time, he had a loaded handgun and was threatening to kill himself and his ex-girlfriend. The patient reported that he had been experiencing extensive depressive symptomatology for 2 months since the breakup of their relationship. Specifically, he reported persistent depressed mood, anhedonia, weight loss of 20 pounds, insomnia, some agitation, poor energy and fatigue, feelings of worthlessness, and diminished attention/concentration, as well as persistent daily suicidal thoughts. In terms of suicidal ideation, he reported thinking of shooting himself as frequent as 10 to 15 times a day. He reported the thoughts as overwhelming; he had purchased a weapon and acted on the thoughts by going over to his ex-girlfriend's house where he was arrested. At the time of his arrest, he was acutely intoxicated and reported that he had been drinking heavily for the past 2 months. He stated that he had been "drunk" everyday for the past 2 weeks. As a result, he recently lost his job. When questioned about intent, the patient stated, "When I get out of here I'm going to kill myself the second I walk out of the door." The patient reported a previous history of suicidal behavior, with an overdose attempt at the age of 18 and a second at 20. Both required acute hospitalization, but he declined further psychiatric treatment. He reported no supportive resources, with strained relationships with his parents and siblings. He stated, "I haven't talked to them in 2 years."

- *Risk category:* Chronic high risk with acute exacerbation.
- *Risk indicators: Category I:* Previous psychiatric history, prior attempts requiring medical care, chaotic family history. *Category II:* Multiple losses (several relationships and job) and family instability. *Category III:* Diagnosis of recurrent major depressive disorder, alcohol dependence, and likely personality disorder. Current symptomatology severe. Significant anger and agitation. Category IV: Marked hopelessness. *Category V:* Frequent, specific, and intense ideation. Available means with active behavior. Clear markers of explicit and implicit intent. No identifiable deterrents. *Category VI:* Multiple attempts, potentially lethal requiring medical care. No help seeking and subsequent help negation. *Category VII:* Marked impulsivity, both subjective and objective. Active substance abuse. *Category VIII:* No identifiable protective factors.
- *Severity rating:* 10. Indicated response: Immediate hospitalization, involuntary if necessary.
- *Treatment response:* Hospitalization to reduce dysphoria, hopelessness, and associated suicidality. Additionally, detoxification for alcohol dependence, control of impulsivity, mobilization of social support system if possible, and initiate establishing an individual psychotherapeutic relationship.

Although brief, the vignette highlights risk variables from each of the eight assessment categories presented earlier. Accordingly, clinical documentation in this case would result in *open* (i.e., rated as greater than 1) risk markers from each category. As a result, each *open* marker would need to be addressed in all subsequent clinical contacts and monitored closely, and the treatment plan would need to be tailored to meet each risk marker. In addition, each risk marker would need to be consistently addressed until each marker was successfully *closed* (i.e., rated as 1 or none). For example, the patient presented with an alcohol dependency problem. The status of his alcohol abuse, participation in a treatment program, and its role in relationship to his suicide risk would need to be actively monitored and documented until effectively resolved (i.e., cessation of all alcohol use). This is perhaps most easily accomplished by incorporation of a standard suicide risk assessment section into all clinical entries. The component parts of such an entry are provided in the previous example (i.e., risk category, risk indicators across each assessment category, severity rating, and treatment response).

If suicide risk is minimal, these entries are brief and subsequent entries need only note that *risk is minimal and unchanged since last assessment.* As markers of risk emerge, they simply need to be *opened*, assessed, and monitored over time until they resolve and once again are effectively *closed.* As is evident, there should be agreement between the patient's suicide risk assessment section and the subsequent treatment plan (e.g., the treatment plan should evidence specific steps [such as medication] to address severe and debilitating depressive symptomatology or recurrent and severe panic attacks). Use of the risk monitoring card provided can streamline the process and provide an easily accessible summary for detailing the suicide risk assessment entry in the clinical chart. This section in the chart can easily be expanded as needed, incorporating a section for professional consultations, telephone monitoring, medication checks, and family involvement, among a host of other variables.

The Role of Chronicity and Time in Risk Assessment

Suicide risk assessment is complicated by the issue of time in two ways. First, identifiable risk periods are inconsistently defined in the literature. Second, chronic suicidality or what Maris (1991) has referred to as suicidal careers complicates estimates of risk. Accordingly, there is general confusion in clinical practice as to what variables are important in risk assessment over relatively short, but clinically relevant, periods (e.g., hours, days, and weeks). It is recommended that risk assessment be a continuous and routine task throughout the course of treatment, with clinical response depending directly on designated category and assessed severity. Risk will naturally vacillate, with periodic acute exacerbation, as ideation, intent, self-control, stressors, and protective factors vary over time.

Clinical Decision Making, Management, and Treatment

A distinct risk assessment scheme will ideally translate into straightforward, clinically indicated, and effective decisions. Figure 6.4 provides a summary of risk categories and indicated clinical responses or options. The standard of care in the management of those at extreme and severe suicide risk is not open for debate, demanding immediate evaluation for inpatient hospitalization (i.e., voluntary or involuntary depending on the circumstances). On the other hand, outpatient management of those at moderate (and possibly severe) risk for suicide can be accomplished safely and effectively and has recently been documented in the literature (e.g., Linehan, 1993; Rudd, Rajab, et al., 1996). If a moderate-risk patient is managed on an outpatient basis, a number of ongoing considerations need to be addressed in the treatment plan until risk subsides: (1) recurrent evaluation of the need for hospitalization; (2) increase in fre-

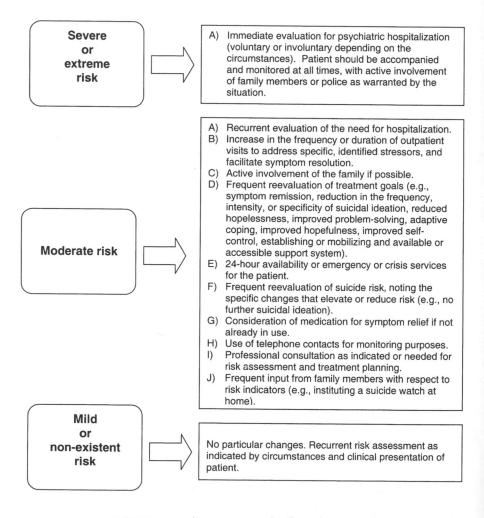

FIGURE 6.4. Risk categories and indicated responses.

quency or duration of outpatient visits; (3) active involvement of the family; (4) frequent reevaluation of treatment plan goals (e.g., symptom remission, reduction in frequency, intensity, duration, or specificity of suicidal ideation, reduced hopelessness, improved problem solving/adaptive coping, improved hopefulness, improved self-control, and establishing/mobilizing an available and accessible support system); (5) 24-hour availability of emergency or crisis services for the patient; (6) frequent reevaluation of suicide risk, noting the specific changes that reduce or elevate risk (e.g., no continuing suicidal ideation, improved social support following reconciliation in a relationship, and improved problem solving); (7) consideration of medication if symptomatology persists or worsen; (8) use of telephone contacts; (9) frequent input from family members with respect to risk indicators (e.g., instituting *suicide watch* at home); and (10) professional consultation as needed or indicated. Those determined to be at mild risk require no particular change in ongoing treatment aside from ensuring recurrent evaluation of any expressed suicidal ideation to determine whether there has been escalation or decline in risk.

Clinical decision making and the management of suicidality are surprisingly straightforward if an accurate risk assessment is completed. Both are simply functions of the limited options available for outpatient management, as well as of the sole option of hospitalization (or extended residential care) under severe or extreme risk. Of importance, a growing body of literature has demonstrated that outpatient management and treatment can be accomplished in a safe and clinically effective manner (Linehan, 1993; Rudd, Rajab, et al., 1996), debunking some of the more persistent myths about working with suicidal patients.

Ongoing Monitoring of Treatment Outcome and Evaluation

As has been discussed previously, monitoring treatment outcome is vital to effective and efficient care. The clinician can monitor treatment outcome by considering both direct and indirect markers of suicidality. Suicide and suicide-related behaviors are just that, behaviors. Accordingly, the only *direct* marker of suicidality is, by definition, a behavioral outcome. In accordance with the framework provided by O'Carroll et al. (1996), behavioral outcomes include suicide attempts and instrumental behaviors. As illustrated in Figure 6.5, both can be further categorized as *with* or *without* injuries. Consistent with the conceptual framework for suicidality offered earlier, indirect markers encompass associated symptoms, identified skill deficits, and maladaptive traits. Clearly, all are related to the patient's specific presentation and need to be monitored throughout the entirety of treatment, regardless of whether or not it is short or long term.

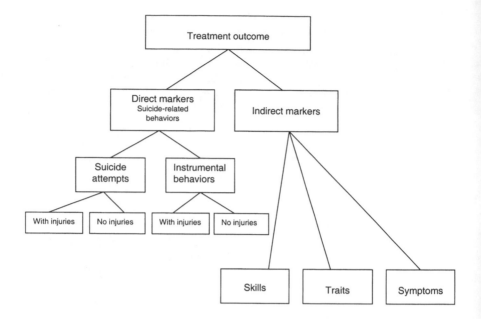

FIGURE 6.5. Conceptualizing treatment outcome.

In an effort to facilitate outcome monitoring, the clinician is encouraged to either use or develop a monitoring sheet such as that illustrated previously in Figure 5.1. The one provided is comprehensive and straightforward and uses simple global clinician ratings to track and organize the patient's progress. The form provided can be modified to fit the needs of a particular clinician or setting. Other assessment instruments can be used for a more precise assessment of symptom intensity (e.g., the Beck Depression Inventory, Beck Anxiety Inventory, and Beck Scale for Suicide Ideation), with a place for summary scores integrated into the monitoring sheet. The form provided can be used in conjunction with those discussed in other chapters. Regardless of whether the clinician chooses to use the form provided, modify it, or develop his or her own, it is important that he or she keep in mind several points about monitoring treatment outcome:

- A standard form should be used for treatment outcome monitoring, particularly if more than one clinician is treating suicidality in the same setting as part of a treatment team.
- The form must be comprehensive in nature, covering both direct and indirect markers of suicidality.

- The form must be fairly simple. Its purpose is to provide an easily accessible summary.
- The form should be completed on a predictable schedule, at least every month, if treatment is short term. If treatment endures for more than 12 months, it should be completed at least every 6 months.
- The monitoring forms should be kept as a part of the permanent clinical record.
- The monitoring forms should be reviewed periodically. This is something that should be a standard practice of the treatment team.

The importance of monitoring treatment outcome cannot be overstated. We have provided what we hope is a simple and straightforward conceptual model for accomplishing this goal. The only risk of monitoring treatment outcome is improving the overall quality and nature of care provided.

The Persistence of Suicidal Thoughts: A Potentially Misleading Marker of Treatment Outcome

It important to recognize that the frequency, specificity, intensity, and duration of suicidal thinking will not always be good markers for treatment outcome, depending on the patient's diagnostic presentation. Frequently, suicidal thinking will diminish and disappear in concert with associated behaviors. For personality disturbed patients and those with complex comorbidity, however, this is not always the case. They may continue to ideate frequently and for long periods. A better marker of progress is the behavioral outcome, that is, whether the patient actually makes a suicide attempt or engages in other self-destructive behaviors.

7

Crisis Intervention and Initial Symptom Management

Slaikeu (1990) defined crisis as "a temporary state of upset and disorganization, characterized chiefly by an individual's inability to cope with a particular situation using customary methods of problem solving" (p. 15). As reviewed in Chapter 6, no two suicidal crises are identical. In an effort to capture some of the qualitative differences in crises, a distinction was made between symptom stabilization, symptom self-management, and symptom utilization during periods of acute suicidal crisis. As discussed, crises vary not only between individuals but also for the same patient over time, particularly during the course of treatment. As treatment progresses, direct intervention on the part of the clinician would hopefully be less frequent and the duration and intensity of crises would lessen.

The crisis presentation can run the full gamut, from episodic, nonspecific suicidal thoughts to a first-time attempt of low lethality to the chronic multiple attempter with recurrent, highly lethal suicide attempts, all requiring intensive medical care. All these clinical presentations are, however, characterized by acute upset and varying degrees of disorganization. Regardless of the specific clinical presentation and consistent with the definition offered by Slaikeu (1990), the suicidal crisis denotes one undeniable truth; the individual sitting in the clinician's office considering or espousing suicide is evidencing an *inability to cope* during an acute (i.e., transient) state. Ultimately, the individual will feel better. For some this will happen in a matter of hours; for others it may take days, weeks, or months. Whether the crisis is the patient's first or only one in a habitual pattern of behavior that spans years, common clinical features need to be identified and addressed to facilitate effective resolution of the crisis and to lay a productive foundation for continuing psychotherapy.

There is a complex and initially confusing web of factors that have led the suicidal patient to the clinician's office. Often, the patient will present with limited understanding, insight, or awareness as to the specific nature of the problem, something not particularly surprising during the early stages of treatment. The confusion characteristic of a dysphoric state is evidenced by the following description spontaneously offered by an acutely suicidal patient (during the initial session):

> "I really didn't know what I was doing. I got the gun out, looked at. I don't really remember thinking. I put a few bullets in it, pointed to my head and just sat there. All I know is that I just wanted to die . . . I wanted all this to end. I pointed it at the floor and pulled the trigger. The noise made me jump. I don't know, it was like it just woke me up. I don't remember if I meant to pull the trigger. It was like it just happened. I had been thinking about it for so long. I got really scared and called, Tina, a friend. That's how I ended up calling you."

Shneidman (1993) referred to this acute dysphoria as *perturbation,* noting that perturbation "refers to how upset (disturbed, agitated, sane–insane, discomposed) the individual is" (p. 138). Shneidman (1993) went on to note that suicide is essentially a function of *perturbation* and *lethality* (i.e., how likely the individual is to take his or her own life).

Key Tasks of Crisis Intervention

The key therapeutic response during a state of suicidal crisis is to detail a specific *crisis response plan* to resolve the acute emotional upset. Although it may sound somewhat concrete, it is important from the very outset to discuss with the patient the criteria for a crisis. In other words, what type of crisis necessitates the use of the crisis response plan? Is it any time the patient thinks about suicide? We recommend that the definition used with patients be similar to that offered earlier. A suicidal crisis is characterized not by simple suicidal thoughts but by associated feelings of hopelessness *and* helplessness to cope in an effective manner. A suicidal crisis, then, occurs when an individual has specific suicidal thoughts that co-occur with acute dysphoria and emotional upset and the individual believes that he or she may act on those thoughts. The crisis response plan should include three critical components, which are the focus of this chapter:

1. The patient needs help in recognizing what triggered the suicidal cri-sis and improving his or her understanding of associated thoughts (i.e., the suicidal belief system) and feelings.
2. The patient needs to intervene in a manner that will work to deacti-vate the suicidal mode and facilitates emotional recovery (i.e., im-prove distress tolerance and emotion regulation skills).
3. If the suicidal mode is not successfully deactivated, the patient needs to access emergency care and assistance in a manner that facilitates skill development and minimizes dependency and manipulation.

The patient's external world will not realistically change to any great de-gree over a session or two, but the sense of emotional urgency and dysphoria, or perturbation, may effectively resolve with *active and specific* intervention. A crisis response plan should include therapeutic responsiveness and flexibil-ity, targeting specifically the patient's sense of hopelessness and helplessness, immediate symptom resolution, guaranteeing the patient's safety, active prob-lem solving, and marshalling supportive resources. Such a plan will, in all likelihood, lower risk and allow a return to more traditional psychotherapy. This is the distinctive feature of a suicidal crisis—acute and intense emotional upset, dysphoria, or perturbation.

In responding to the crisis, it is important for the clinician to recognize and differentiate between an episodic or acute crisis with high intent from re-current, and potentially habitual, suicidal crises with low intent. As discussed in Chapter 6, a distinction needs to be made between chronic multiple at-tempters and all others (i.e., ideators, and single attempters). Although early in the treatment process all crises will be handled in a similar fashion (i.e., a probable assumption of high intent), the therapeutic focus and treatment tar-gets will likely vary for multiple attempters as the therapeutic relationship is firmly established and the suicidal mode is better understood (see Chapter 8). As illustrated in Figure 7.1, there are some potentially important distinctions between chronic or habitual crises with low intent and acute suicidal crises with high intent.

It is important to point out that the differences discussed are only *poten-tial differences*. This does not, by any means, imply that all multiple attempt-ers have motivations *other* than suicide. To the contrary, some of our own work has clearly demonstrated the undeniably high-risk nature of multiple at-tempters (Rudd, Joiner, & Rajab, 1996). Also, as was discussed in Chapter 6, those who have made multiple attempts are essentially at chronic high risk and can experience acute exacerbation. For effective treatment of this chronic pop-ulation, however, it is critical to adequately assess and treat this issue of intent in some capacity.

As illustrated in Figure 7.1 and described in Chapter 2, the suicidal mode

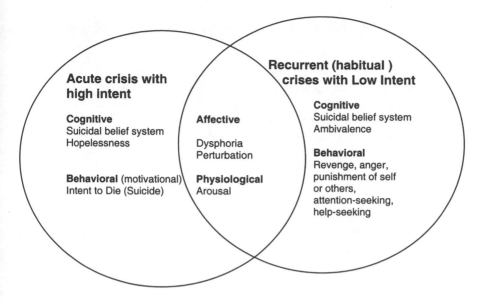

Acute crisis with
high intent

Cognitive
Suicidal belief system
Hopelessness

Behavioral (motivational)
Intent to Die (Suicide)

Affective

Dysphoria
Perturbation

Physiological
Arousal

Recurrent (habitual)
crises with Low Intent

Cognitive
Suicidal belief system
Ambivalence

Behavioral
Revenge, anger,
punishment of self
or others,
attention-seeking,
help-seeking

FIGURE 7.1. The characteristic features of crises with low and high intent.

varies in accordance with its component parts: cognitive, affective, behavioral, and physiological. During an acute suicidal crisis, regardless of whether or not it is indicative of a habitual pattern (with low intent) or an episodic problem (with high intent), the patient will manifest acute emotional upset and physiological arousal. For the multiple attempter with chronic suicidality, however, the possibility of distinctive motivational or behavioral features needs to considered and weighed. This does not in any way mean that ideators or single attempters cannot present with a motivation other than death, or that a multiple attempter does not at times clearly intend on dying by suicide.* It simply relates that an individual with habitual suicidal crises is more likely to have other motivations and purposes than death, particularly the longer the behavior persists. Most frequently, such motivations include anger, revenge, punishment of self or others, inappropriate or inadequate help seeking, or attention seeking. Most important, though, the clinician must be aware of the possibility of other motivations and monitor it throughout the treatment process. The motivation and purpose for the behavior are critical to eliminating suicidality during the course of treatment (see Chapter 8). Also, as indicated in Figure 7.1,

---

*This is stated simply to denote the importance of the behavioral/motivational component of the suicidal mode for ongoing treatment.

during acute crises with high intent, the suicidal belief system is characterized by overt hopelessness. For those experiencing habitual crises with low intent, the suicidal belief system is likely to be characterized by marked ambivalence. The differences noted in both the suicidal belief system and the motivational/behavioral systems for acute crises with high intent versus habitual crises with low intent are critical for effective and efficient ongoing care.

When someone presents in a state of acute dysphoria, is *perturbed* and suicidal, regardless of the duration of treatment, it will constrain (appropriately so) the very nature of the interventions being used. The acute dysphoria and perturbation demand immediate attention. As summarized by Shneidman (1993) and others (e.g., Bongar, 1991; Slaikeu, 1990), crisis intervention and initial symptom management need to attend to some specific goals. This chapter provides a general summary of the goals for crisis intervention and initial symptom management, followed by a more detailed discussion of each, along with a few clinical examples. It is important to note that it may well take several sessions (i.e., 1–4 most frequently) to accomplish the goals listed, depending on the patient's particular clinical presentation. Also, the primary focus of crisis intervention and initial symptom management is to generate a *crisis response plan* incorporating the three component parts referenced earlier. Although there may be others, the most salient tasks of crisis intervention include the following:

• Ensure the safety of the patient. Remove any available or accessible means of suicide. In accordance with the discussion of risk assessment issues in Chapter 5, this will require careful, methodical, and thorough questioning, along with the necessary and indicated responses (e.g., securing a gun, close supervision of medications for a limited time, and home monitoring by family or friends).

• Initiate self-monitoring, particularly during periods of acute emotional upset (i.e., improve the patient's awareness and understanding of his or her own cognitive, emotional, and behavioral functioning—the patient's *suicidal mode*). As discussed in detail later, self-monitoring can be initiated in a relatively simple and straightforward fashion. Often, it can simply be integrated into the assessment process.

• Target and achieve symptom remission and stabilization (i.e., the *most disruptive* symptoms). It is important to identify and target those symptoms the patient identifies as *most disruptive*. In other words, what symptoms are impairing the patient's ability to function on a day-to-day basis (e.g., insomnia, panic, and agitation)?

• Target the *source* of the patient's hopelessness directly (e.g., a particular precipitating event, relationship, circumstance, or situation). In targeting the patient's *source hopelessness*, active problem solving will be necessary (see Chapter 10). In the end, the patient's options may not be greatly expanded, but if the patient recognizes that there is at least one option better than suicide, that may be enough.

• Initiate immediate activity, regardless of its significance, to undermine the patient's sense of helplessness. In other words, it is important to *do something*, but it needs to be something strategic, specific, and consistent with the longer-term treatment plan and directed at the patient's source hopelessness.

• Marshall support to undermine the patient's sense of isolation and detachment, involving family, friends, or significant other as needed or indicated.

• Identify (and clarify) the patient's *active* suicidal mode, with a particular focus on the cognitive and behavioral (motivational) components. In addition to targeting the patient's *source hopelessness* directly, the suicidal belief system (cognitive component) and motivational component of the suicidal mode are ripe targets for intervention during acute crisis.

• Identify the patient's most profound skill deficits, that is, those associated with the suicidal crisis. What is it that the patient is having trouble doing (e.g., regulating emotion effectively, asserting him or herself in a relationship, tolerating distress, or expressing anger in a constructive manner)? What is the patient doing to make the problem(s) worse (e.g., substance abuse)? What is the patient doing well that he or she may not readily recognize or actively dismiss?

• Provide a crisis response plan. It is important for the patient to have a clearly articulated, specific *crisis/emergency response plan*, one that attributes as much responsibility to the patient as possible.

• Articulate (and modify as needed) the initial conceptual model for intervention, that is, the *suicidal cycle*.

• Reinforce the patient's commitment to treatment as a preferable alternative to suicide. This is something that can be done repeatedly throughout a session, often in subtle but important ways.

• Solidify the therapeutic relationship by maintaining flexibility and availability and being responsive to the patient's identified needs. As discussed in Chapter 9, the therapeutic relationship is the cornerstone of treatment. Careful monitoring and management of the therapeutic belief system (see Chapter 9) are critical for effective treatment.

Ensuring the Patient's Safety

As has been noted by Shneidman (1993) and Bongar (1991), among many others, a primary goal in a suicidal crisis is to simply *keep the person alive*. To effectively do this, we need to ensure the patient's safety. As detailed in Chapter 6, clinical decision making is directly linked to the patient's identified risk category. During acute suicidal crises the following steps need to be taken:

- If there is clear expressed intent, there needs to be immediate referral for psychiatric evaluation and consideration for hospitalization. Under these conditions, the patient should be accompanied and monitored at all times, with active involvement of family members or police as warranted by the situation.
- Regardless of risk category, it is important to remove access to or availability of means of suicide (e.g., gun or medications—which should be closely monitored during crises perhaps with coordination of family members).
- If the patient does not express clear intent and will continue to be treated on an outpatient basis, then the recommendations in Chapter 6 for managing someone at moderate risk need to be followed.

Self-Monitoring *during* Crises

It is important to introduce structure in some form or fashion during a crisis state. As discussed earlier, an active suicidal mode is characterized by hopeless cognitions and intense feelings of helplessness and dysphoria. A structured intervention provides the patient a means to (1) diffuse or *deactivate* the suicidal mode, (2) inhibit intensification of emotion, (3) develop some very basic skills, (4) alter the hopeless nature of the suicidal belief system, and (5) provide a foundation necessary for lasting personality development. The easiest and most efficient way to intervene is with the suicidal thought record, along with subjective ratings of symptoms and feelings (see Figure 7.2). The ultimate goal is to use the STR and subjective ratings to illustrate the suicidal cycle, identifying specifically for the patient the necessary points for intervention and change.

There are three identifiable goals with respect to improving self-monitoring (as detailed in Chapter 3). First, it is important for patients simply to become more aware (i.e., label) of what they are feeling and thinking. Second, they need to accurately understand (i.e., normalize the feelings within the current crisis context) their feelings. And third, they need to learn to respond to them (i.e., express and regulate) more effectively. Development of these specific skills is discussed in detail in Chapter 10. Next we review several techniques or tools to facilitate self-monitoring during periods of acute crisis.

Teaching the Patient to Rate Discomfort:
A Self-Monitoring Task

Completing an STR during the early stages of an acute crisis session may not be practical (see Figure 7.2). The clinician needs to be sensitive to the fact that use of both the STR and depicting the patient's suicidal cycle is recommended

Triggering event(s)[A]	Suicidal thoughts[B]	Severity[C] (1–10)	Duration[D] (1–10)	Feelings[E]	Severity (1–10)	Duration (1–10)	Behavioral response[F]	Change[G] +/–
Friday, July 3, 1998, 7:35 P.M. My boyfriend left after an argument, it was just me and him. I was at home alone.	I thought about taking an overdose of my antidepressant. The pills were in my purse.	9	20 minutes.	Anger, frustration, sadness.	9	About 15 minutes.	I went and listened to some music, thought about drinking a beer but didn't.	++

FIGURE 7.2. Example of a completed Suicidal Thought Record/self-monitoring sheet.

[A]Provide as much detail as possible. Indicate the full context, what day, time, who was present, what happened, and what did you do?
[B]Describe the specific thought(s) you had at the time. For example, "I thought of taking an overdose, that I didn't deserve to live, everybody would be better off if I was dead."
[C]Describe the intensity or severity of your thoughts on a scale of 1–10, with 1 being mild and 10 overwhelming.
[D]Note how long the thoughts lasted, a few seconds, minutes, hours, or days. Please try to be precise.
[E]Describe your feelings such as anger, sadness, guilt, anxiety. Remember, you can feel more than one thing at a time.
[F]Describe what you did in response to the trigger and your suicidal thoughts. Remember, doing nothing is doing something!
[G]Please indicate any change in your thoughts or how you felt as a result of your behavioral response, just note it as positive (+) or negative (–).

155

only after the most intense dysphoria and upset have been effectively diffused. On occasion, this may take several sessions. By the end of the first or second session, however, it can be relatively easy for the clinician to complete the STR *with* the patient. The STR can then be used to depict the suicidal cycle, providing a concise and clear summary of the crisis for the patient. It is recommended that the clinician actually take out a sheet of paper (or use a blackboard) and draw the cycle, clearly depicting the various points for intervention consistent with the articulated treatment plan. As discussed in more detail later, this provides remarkable structure and clarity to a situation previously characterized as *chaotic and disorganized.* As a result, the clinician often hears patients say, "I finally understand what's going on with me." This is a critical thing, helping the patient become more aware of behavioral patterns and also improving his or her understanding of typical *suicidal cycles.*

Self-monitoring can be accomplished simply by having the patient articulate *subjective ratings* (e.g., ranging from 1 to 10) of various feelings and symptoms (consistent with the assessment framework provided in Chapter 6) periodically throughout the session(s). Initiating self-monitoring in this way provides an opportunity to accomplish a number of subtle but important tasks. First, it introduces structure and predictable organization to treatment. That is, it makes it clear that a consistent therapeutic task is to monitor the intensity of emotions and related symptomatology over time. As a result, it provides a sense of control, power, or influence for the patient. Third, it provides a means to target the patient's sense of hopelessness and helplessness in a direct fashion. During an acute suicidal crisis, patients often voice that their *feelings will never end or change* and that they *cannot tolerate them.* Statements like this demonstrate both a hopelessness about the patient's current emotional turmoil as well as a related sense of helplessness to do anything about it. Implementing self-monitoring by using subjective ratings demonstrates for patients that they can directly influence, and modify in a constructive manner, the intensity of their emotional experience. Sometimes the changes can be fairly dramatic over the course of a 45- to 50-minute session. The following vignette demonstrates such a change over a relatively brief period.

PATIENT: I just can't stand it anymore. It's the last time I'm going to let him do that to me. I'm just so hurt and ticked off. All I can think about is finally killing myself. I don't ever want to feel like this again.

THERAPIST: You really sound angry and hurt about what happened, can you help me get a better idea of just how angry and hurt you are? Could you rate it on a scale from one to ten, with ten being the most angry you've ever felt?

PATIENT: Oh, I'd say it's a ten. I really feel like I need to do something to hurt him. But I can't so I just want to kill myself.

THERAPIST [toward the end of the same session]: We've been talking now for about thirty minutes or so. You don't sound as angry, hurt, or upset. Could you rate your anger again on a scale of one to ten?

PATIENT: Huh? I think you might be right. Since we've been talking about some things I can do, I really don't feel as angry. I'd say it's about a seven or eight now.

THERAPIST: If that's true, It'd seem like something you said a little bit earlier may not necessarily be true. Earlier you said you didn't think you'd ever stop feeling the way you did when you came in.

PATIENT: You might be right. I do feel better right now, not a bunch, but I can tell a difference.

THERAPIST: What have we done to make that possible?

PATIENT: We really haven't done that much. We've talked about what's going on and maybe a few things I can do differently.

THERAPIST: So, would it be fair to say that you can reduce your anger by expressing it in a constructive way and problem solving a little?

PATIENT: Yeah, I guess it would.

THERAPIST: What do you usually do when you get this mad?

PATIENT: I usually drink . . . a lot.

THERAPIST: What usually happens when you drink a lot?

PATIENT: I guess I end up throwing stuff around the apartment. The last couple of times I ended up cutting my wrists.

THERAPIST: It sounds like those steps only make things worse. Here, we did a few things differently that helped. We talked about it, gave you an outlet, and considered a few other options and your anger subsided, actually by as much as 20% in only a half hour.

As evidenced by this passage, acutely suicidal patients are, often, unaware of the natural changes in emotional intensity over time. In short, the idea that if they *just wait a little while they might feel better* is lost. Also, as is apparent in the passage, their pervasive sense of hopelessness and helplessness can cloud any sense of influence or control they might exert (e.g., simple appropriate emotional expression and problem solving). Finally, suicidal patients are often unaware of the steps they may be actively taking that only intensify, rather than diminish, their dysphoria and upset.

Completing the Suicidal Thought Record

Once the patient is familiar with subjective ratings of emotional upset and dysphoria, this information can be translated directly to the STR (see Figure 7.2). Completing the STR is a relatively easy and straightforward process (going from Box *A–G* in the figure):

1. Identify the triggering event(s). Provide as much detail as possible. Indicate the full context for the triggering event(s). What are the patient's reasons for dying? Why does the patient want to die right now? What day was it? What time? Who was present? What happened? And, finally, what did the patient do?
2. Describe the specific suicidal thoughts the patient voiced. How does the patient describe him- or herself when actively suicidal? How does the patient describe others? Be as detailed as possible. It is not uncommon for the intent of the thought to change when the patient is specific. For example, it is not uncommon for a patient to say, "I didn't really think about killing myself at first, I just wanted to stop hurting," and add later, "I only started thinking about suicide after I drank." This detail indicates a two-step process rather than immediate onset of suicidality during a crisis and can be very important in articulating the crisis response plan.
3. Have the patient rate the severity or intensity of the thoughts on a scale of 1–10.
4. Have the patient estimate the duration of the thoughts. Again, it is important to be as specific as possible. Was it a few seconds, a few minutes, hours, days? Ultimately, markers of severity and duration of suicidal thoughts will provide insight into recovery.
5. Have the patient describe *all* relevant feelings, such as depression, sadness, anger, guilt, or anxiety. Always remind patients that they can feel more than one thing at a time.
6. Have patients describe what they did in response to the triggering event and the subsequent suicidal thoughts. What does the patient believe will help him or her feel better? Again, remind patients that *doing nothing* is *doing something*.
7. Finally, have the patient indicate any change in his or her thoughts or feelings as a result of his or her behavioral response. This change can simply be denoted as positive (+) or negative (–) in the appropriate column of the STR.

Once the STR is completed it can be used to depict the suicidal cycle. The STR is, however, an important self-monitoring tool in its own right.

Depicting the Suicidal Cycle: The Suicidal Mode in Action

All the previous steps help make the patient's crisis understandable in very concrete terms—terms that translate easily into the treatment goals and targets summarized in Chapter 3. An essential component of time-limited treatment is that it must be understandable; the tools and techniques used must be understood as important and accepted as effective by the patient. Essentially, the process of depicting the patient's *suicidal cycle* integrates what, at times, can be disparate and confusing information discussed during a session. The suicidal cycle is simply the *suicidal mode in action*. It provides an effective summary of the crisis intervention session and lends itself to a discussion of specific treatment goals and targets, particularly over the short term. For example, at the end of the session the therapist might say the following:

> "We've talked about quite a few things today. You've described a broad range of thoughts, feelings, and a few things that you've done in response. But, I think the most significant thing we've talked about is that you've been thinking that the only alternative to your current problems is to suicide. Let's try to organize things a bit. Let's see if we can put all of this down into a conceptual model that might help us better understand exactly what the problems are, where you're getting stuck, and the things that we need to be working on over the next few weeks."

The suicidal cycle can be completed by answering and organizing a few straightforward questions that can be taken directly from the STR (see Figure 7.3):

- What triggered the crisis?
- What were the patient's suicidal thoughts?
- What were they feeling?
- What physical symptoms were present?
- What was the behavioral response?
- What was the motivation (i.e., death, or something else)?

As detailed in Chapter 3, Ms. D responded to her suicidal cycle with, "That's me! I can't believe we could put it down on paper like that." Another patient would frequently refer to his conceptual model with "Every time something triggers a suicidal thought, I get a picture of that model in my head and it makes it easier for me to think about what I need to do to feel better." We have found that depicting the patient's suicidal crises in concrete terms has not only been effective in clinical terms but also is well received by patients. Of critical

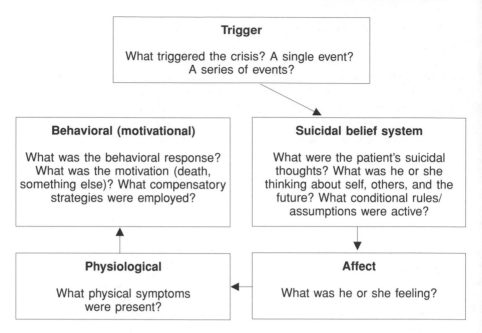

FIGURE 7.3. The suicidal mode in action: Questions to answer in completing the suicidal cycle.

importance is that the suicidal cycle summarizes the treatment agenda in simple and concise format. Each step in the cycle is a treatment target and, taken all together, the steps comprise the treatment agenda. It is an easy and straightforward way to convey to the patient what psychotherapy for suicidal behavior involves.

Using Mood Graphs

The mood graph illustrated in Figure 7.4 is particularly useful for patients who have limited self-monitoring skills, limited awareness of natural mood fluctuations, and a pervasive sense of helplessness (e.g., "I'll always feel this way, there's nothing I can do"). The graph can be used over a period of hours (e.g., 12- to 24-hour time frames), days, or months depending on the identified goal. We recommend the use of mood graphs for patients who have trouble identifying mood fluctuations when completing the STR. It is easiest to use for a specified number of hours, a single day, or a period of a few days. All that is needed to complete a mood graph is to have the patient keep a *mood log* over

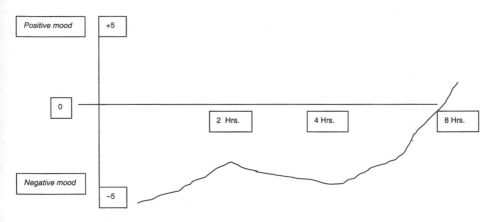

FIGURE 7.4. Example of a mood graph.

the period of a few hours or a day or two. Patients simply need to rate their mood on a scale of 1–10 at various points during they day. To facilitate ease of use, we have patients rate their mood at breakfast, lunch, dinner, and bedtime. They can use an index card or a small tablet that they can carry in either their shirt pocket or purse.

Once the clinician has the ratings, he or she can sit down with the patient and translate the ratings to a mood graph (see Figure 7.4). It is easiest for patients to understand if the clinician distinguishes between negative and positive mood. Therefore, the clinician can translate the 1–10 scale to a –5 to +5 scale, drawing a line across the middle to indicate an unremarkable or indifferent mood (i.e., 0 on the scale in the figure). By graphing the various ratings over the period of specified hours or a day and then simply connecting the dots, the clinician can demonstrate for the patient that his or her moods do in fact fluctuate, although sometimes in subtle ways.

As illustrated, the clinician simply needs to adjust the time frame indicated on the graph in accordance with the time period targeted. If the clinician is targeting a period of hours, the x-axis will be hours; if he or she is targeting days, it will be days. It is most useful, however, to use the mood graph as a means of monitoring mood changes and fluctuations over relatively short periods, perhaps a few hours or a single day. This helps the patient recognize the critical lesson that *bad feelings do not last forever.* In fact, patients will come to understand that feelings routinely change quite a bit in a morning or afternoon. In addition to completing the graph, it is important for the clinician to review the graph with the patient, identifying not only fluctuations in mood but also behaviors, events, and circumstances that may have influenced or corresponded with mood changes. It is important for the patient to clearly recognize the presence of not only destructive and self-defeating behaviors but also those that serve a productive and stabilizing influence.

Improving Distress Tolerance and Reducing Impulsivity: The Importance of Repeatedly Emphasizing That Bad Feelings Do Not Last Forever

As Shneidman (1993) stated, "suicide is the human act of self-inflicted, self-intended cessation (i.e., the permanent stopping of consciousness)" (p. 137). The goal is not always death but frequently a simple desire to stop feeling so badly. For many suicidal patients the simple fact that *bad feelings do not last forever* gets lost in the morass of pain, hurt, guilt, and dysphoria. One of the primary goals of crisis intervention is to help the patient improve his or her overall *distress tolerance*. It is critical that patients learn this simple but powerful lesson. In addition, treatment can help patients recognize that not only do bad feelings not endure forever, but they can take identifiable steps to actively facilitate their own recovery.

As Linehan (1993) has aptly noted, poor distress tolerance and impulsivity are inextricably intertwined. Impulsive behaviors (e.g., substance abuse, self-cutting/self abuse, aggressiveness, sexual acting out, and suicidal behaviors) frequently occur in an effort to relieve intense emotional hurt and pain, not necessarily to suicide. Similarly, suicide becomes an option if the patient believes the emotional pain resultant from a precipitating event (or chronic problems) can no longer be reasonably endured. As discussed in more detail in Chapter 10, poor distress tolerance is characterized by a low threshold for reaction, extreme reactivity, and prolonged recovery (e.g., Linehan, 1993).

During periods of acute crisis, each of these deficits can be targeted directly. This is best done by implementing the self-monitoring techniques referenced earlier. To maximize the opportunity, however, it is critical for the clinician to establish this as a central goal of crisis intervention. Most cognitive-behavioral therapists agree that a necessary condition for therapeutic change is the presence of *hot cognitions*: an active, emotionally charged, accessible, and accordingly modifiable belief system (e.g., Persons, 1995; Rudd & Joiner, 1998a; Safran & Greenberg, 1986). In accordance with the CBT approach recommended here, the suicidal mode and suicidal belief system are most amenable to change during periods of activation, that is, during acute crises. Ensuring that critical beliefs are identified and challenged during periods of crisis is the task of the treating clinician.

Steps for Improving Distress Tolerance

Following is a summary of recommended intervention guidelines:

- Implement self-monitoring early in the crisis, using simple subjective symptom severity rating scales.
- Periodically rate severity of distress, feelings, or overall emotional upset throughout the course of the session(s).
- Clearly identify for the patient any noticeable reductions in emotional upset, even if very subtle (e.g., 1 point), along with any identifiable physiological correlates (e.g., slowing of heart rate and respiration rate).
- Identify and discuss steps the patient took to facilitate recovery and reduce symptomatology.
- Contrast recovery with previous episodes in which the patient may have taken steps that only served to exacerbate symptoms and emotional upset. Be specific as to the role of destructive behaviors (e.g., substance abuse, self-cutting, hitting or throwing things, destroying property, or reinitiating contact with someone with whom the patient was arguing).
- Identify and discuss the implications for any observed changes in terms of the patient's distress tolerance skills. That is, can the patient tolerate more than he or she initially thought? What does this say about the patient's skill level?
- Have the patient draw (and document in his or her journal or treatment log) specific conclusions regarding his or her skills and abilities for crisis and symptom management. For example, a patient concluded the following at the end of a crisis session:

"When I get upset and think about suicide, if I stop and write in my journal, maybe do an STR, go for a walk, or listen to some music, I feel much better after only about thirty minutes passes. Also, I feel much better about myself later on because it helps me learn that I really can handle difficult problems well. I feel more confident in myself. The next day, I'm always glad I didn't kill myself. It scares me how close I've come sometimes."

Targeting Source Hopelessness: A Different Kind of Problem Solving

During periods of acute suicidal crisis, it is important to target the patient's *source hopelessness* in order to diffuse the immediate crisis. This is the precipitating event or circumstance that triggered the patient's suicidality. In other words, what is at the root of the patient's hopelessness during this crisis? Why does the patient want to suicide at this moment? A considerable number of suicidal patients present with pervasive, chronic hopelessness, particularly chronic multiple attempters. More often than not, this pervasive hopelessness is consistent with prominent personality disturbance. Each suicidal crisis will likely, however, be precipitated by an identifiable event, real, imagined, significant, or potentially even trivial (i.e., from an outsider's perspective). Regardless of the nature of the precipitating event, it is important to distinguish between source hopelessness and that which is more chronic in nature and a target of ongoing longer-term treatment. For crisis purposes, it is important to identify and target source hopelessness almost exclusively. This is done by identifying the precipitating event and engaging in problem solving specific to that triggering event. Efforts to expand the problem may only overwhelm the patient during an acute crisis state.

For the majority of patients, identifying source hopelessness will not necessarily be a difficult task. In all likelihood, the patient will readily identify the precipitating event or circumstance. In other words, the patient will come in telling the clinician what the problem is, why the patient wants to kill him- or herself. If not, the self-monitoring steps summarized previously will facilitate the process considerably. In short, clinicians can identify source hopelessness by answering the question, "What triggered the patient's suicidal crisis?" This information is readily available on the STR. It may be a recent relationship loss, argument, job conflict, financial problem, poor performance in a class, illness, or family squabble. Regardless of the nature of the precipitant, active problem solving should be specifically focused in order to effectively diffuse the crisis. Active problem solving is discussed in detail in Chapter 10 but will require the clinician to be active, strategic, organized, and specific in his or her interventions. The following brief vignette provides an example of targeting source hopelessness.

The Case of Mrs. F

The patient, an adult female, presented with prominent symptoms consistent with posttraumatic stress disorder and a comorbid depression after being involved in a motor vehicle accident in which the other driver was killed. She had no prior psychiatric history and, for the most part, had been personally and professionally successful. At the time of the session, the patient presented as acutely suicidal. Tearful and mildly hyperventilating, she stated:

> "I just want to kill myself. I can't stand it anymore. All day I see that women's face, she's screaming. I can't get it out of my mind. I'm a murderer. I feel so guilty for what has happened. Her husband's going to sue me and I think he deserves to win. Last night I got the pistol out and almost shot myself. I just can't take it anymore. I don't deserve to live because I'm just a murderer."

As illustrated, the patient's hopelessness is rooted in her guilt over the accident and death of another person. As noted, she decided she was a *murderer.* This belief provided the foundation for the patient's suicidal belief system. Specifically, she stated, "I don't deserve to live because I'm a murderer" (a conditional rule/assumption; it can be restated as "If I'm a murderer then I don't deserve to live"). Accordingly, this was the focus of the session. The patient was encouraged to define the term "murderer," which eventually led her to the recognition that the precipitant was *an accident* in which she *had no control.* As a result, she was able to redefine both her and the women who had been killed as *victims,* in very different ways but nonetheless both victims of a tragic accident. As expected, this targeted intervention did not entirely alleviate the patient's guilt (her source hopelessness) but enough to diffuse the suicidal crisis and allow the patient to engage in constructive ongoing therapy regarding the grief associated with the accident.

Steps for Targeting Source Hopelessness

To identify and target the patient's source hopelessness during a suicidal crisis, it is important for the clinician to consider a few guiding questions:

- What is the structural content of the patient's suicidal belief system (see Chapter 2)?
- Why does the patient want to die by suicide at this moment?
- What is the meaning attached to the precipitant by the patient?
- What conditional rules/assumptions are operative (i.e., what conditions has the patient established to support his or her suicide)? For example, "If I keep feeling this way then I'll have to kill myself"; "If my husband leaves, I won't be able to survive and then I'll have to kill myself"; "If I lose my job then I'll suicide."
- What are the most prominent symptoms that essentially *fuel* the patient's upset and dysphoria (e.g., insomnia, agitation, anxiety, panic, guilt, and shame)?
- What strategic and concrete steps could be taken to (1) disprove the conditional assumption(s), (2) restructure the meaning associated with the precipitant, and (3) diffuse the most prominent symptoms?

Symptom Matching: Improving Level of Functioning over the Short Term

To facilitate rapid recovery and stabilization, it is important to tailor interventions to the patient's most disruptive symptomatology (i.e., to initiate *symptom matching*). Suicidal patients present with a broad range of symptomatology and comorbidity. Frequently, their breadth and intensity can be confusing and potentially overwhelming for the clinician. We recommend that clinicians identify the symptoms that are the most disruptive to the patient (i.e., those that limit his or her ability to function and are given the highest subjective ratings) and match his or her interventions accordingly. For example, if the patient reports marked insomnia, leading to fatigue and continued decline in functioning, behavioral steps might be taken to improve sleep hygiene or short-term medication might be considered. Similarly, if the patient reports disruptive panic attacks, the clinician might spend time in session on CBT treatment of panic or might consider targeted medications.

Steps for Symptom Matching

To accomplish symptom matching during periods of acute crisis, the following steps are recommended:

- Complete a brief symptom inventory. That is, simply make a list of the patient's most prominent symptoms.
- Have the patient identify the most disruptive symptoms, that is, those that most impair his or her ability to function on a day-to-day basis. This can be done by using subjective ratings or simple descriptions. For the most part, this amounts to creating a symptom matching hierarchy. It is often helpful to simply write the hierarchy on a sheet of paper or blackboard so that it can be more fully considered and modified if needed (see Figure 7.5). As is evident in the figure, insomnia and panic are resulting in the most disruption and impairment and need to be specifically targeted.
- Tailor interventions specifically to those symptoms deemed most disruptive.
- At each successive session, review the symptom hierarchy, modifying it as needed, depending on when symptoms resolve. Also, review the effectiveness of the targeted interventions, continue if effective, modify them as needed if partially effective, or incorporate new ones if entirely ineffective.

The Importance of Structure: Providing a Crisis Response Plan

As noted at the beginning of this chapter, the development of a crisis response plan is critical and the focus of crisis intervention and initial symptom management. During periods of acute crisis, the importance of structure and a specific action plan cannot be overstated. If a clinician is operating under a man-

Symptom(s)	Impairment rating (1–10)/description
Insomnia	10, I've had insomnia for the past 5 days. I haven't been able to sleep more than 3 hours a night and I'm getting really run down. I think it's making my depression worse.
Panic	8, My panic attacks have returned over the last week. As a result I've had to leave work several times and called in sick on two different days.
Guilt	6, I feel really guilty for ending the relationship, but I've felt this way for months now.
Depression	6, My depression is pretty bad and I think it's getting worse because I'm not sleeping.
Shame	5, I still feel ashamed of the abuse that happened but I've felt that way my whole life.
Worry, ruminations	5, I still worry all the time, so what's new.

FIGURE 7.5. Symptom hierarchy.

aged care umbrella and facing time constraints and related limitations, the need for structure takes on added importance. As an acutely suicidal patient wrote in her daily journal, "I entered into a world of unending chaos, a world in which I didn't know the rules anymore." When patients feel this way, structure becomes imperative. All the steps summarized previously provide considerable structure to crisis intervention and initial symptom management. However, one additional area deserves mention.

Coping cards (Beck, 1995) can be extremely useful in delineating a *crisis response plan* for the suicidal patient. Essentially, the coping card is a detailed plan with specific instructions on how to respond to a given situation or circumstance which the patient is to implement during a period of acute suicidal crisis. It is important to write out the plan in some form or fashion. This can be done on a 3 × 5 card, on the back of a business card, or on a sheet of paper. It is important that the coping card be convenient to carry, in either a wallet or a purse. This provides the patient some organization and structure, and a specific series of steps to follow, during periods of acute emotional upset (i.e., when perturbed) when he or she will not be thinking clearly or coherently. Figure 7.6 provides an example of a crisis response plan.

As mentioned previously, the crisis response plan needs to make use of three primary components. First, the patient needs to have an understanding of his or her emotional upset. In other words, what triggered the crisis, why is he or she upset, what is he or she thinking and feeling? Second, the patient needs to respond in a productive manner, working to deactivate the suicidal mode rather than facilitating emotional upset and dysphoria. And, finally, if the patient is not successful in deactivating the suicidal mode, access to emergency care needs to be ensured.

Steps for Creating a Crisis Response Plan

A typical crisis response plan must incorporate the following sequential steps (see Figure 7.6):

1. The patient needs to recognize and understand what events triggered the suicidal crises. Similarly, patients need to know what specific suicidal thoughts and feelings they are experiencing. This is accomplished by use of the STR. Therefore, Step 1 should be to have the patient complete the STR.

2. The patient needs to intervene in a manner that deactivates the suicidal mode and facilitates recovery rather than an escalation of the crisis. This is best communicated by a series of steps. As illustrated on the card in Figure 7.6, intervention can be accomplished by making use of the STR and having the patient implement some basic skills. The three skills of primary importance are cognitive restructuring of the suicidal belief system, distress toler-

---

Crisis response plan: When I'm upset and thinking about suicide, I'll take the following steps.

Step 1. Complete an STR and try to identify specifically what's upsetting me.

Step 2. Write out and review more reasonable responses to my suicidal thoughts, including thoughts about myself, others, and the future.

Step 3. Review all the conclusions I've come to about these thoughts in the past in my treatment log. For example, that the abuse wasn't my fault and I don't have anything to feel ashamed of.

Step 4. Try and do the things that help me feel better for at least 30 minutes (listening to music, going to work out, calling my best friend).

Step 5. Repeat all of the above.

Step 6. If the thoughts continue, get specific, and I find myself preparing to do something, I'll call the emergency call person at (phone number: XXX-XXXX).

Step 7. If I still feel suicidal and don't feel like I can control my behavior, I'll go to the emergency room.

FIGURE 7.6. A sample crisis response plan.

ance, and emotion regulation. It is recommended that the clinician have the patient respond directly to suicidal thoughts (see Chapter 9) with alternative responses (Step 2), reviewing all previous conclusions about specific suicidal thoughts (Step 3), and implement specific activities that reduce emotional upset (Step 4) (i.e., distress tolerance and emotion regulation skills, see Chapter 10). Given that it may take time and effort to diffuse the acute dysphoria and upset, it is advisable to have the patient repeat Steps 1–4 again (Step 5).

3. If the suicidal mode is not successfully deactivated, the patient should access emergency care. It is recommended that a two-tier system be used with the patient accessing the clinician via phone first (Step 6) followed by emergency room care if necessary (Step 7). The goal in using a two-tier system is to maximize independent functioning and reduce utilization of emergency, and possibly inpatient, care as much as possible.

The crisis response plan needs to be specific, detailed in step-by-step fashion (see Figure 7.6). It also needs to be in language understandable to the patient and to include steps that the patient has had input into identifying. Therefore, although such a plan should be developed by both the clinician and the patient, it is best to have the patient actually write it down. The clinician should review the crisis response plan on a regular basis, perhaps every session early in treatment and then maybe once a month later in the treatment process. He or she should modify the plan as needed. If the patient's skills have developed and certain steps are no longer necessary, the clinician should eliminate them. He or she should reinforce the patient for appropriate and effective use of the crisis response plan. Also, the clinician should acknowledge therapeutic progress and success as the impetus for changing the crisis response plan (e.g., when certain steps are no longer necessary).

The use of coping cards for a crisis response plan has a number of advantages. First, coping cards are simple, specific, and effective. Second, the cards are flexible and is designed to meet the needs of the particular patient. Third, they can be modified as patients develop skills and progress during the course of treatment, an issue of particular importance for those manifesting chronic suicidality (see Chapter 8). Fourth, coping cards provide a means for the patient to assume responsibility (as much as is possible) during periods of acute crisis.

This chapter reviews a structured and organized approach to crisis intervention and initial symptom management. Central to effective management of suicidal crises is establishing and developing improved self-monitoring skills. The next chapter covers additional short- and longer-term strategies for reducing suicidal behaviors by learning to intervene and disrupt the suicidal cycle.

8

Reducing and Eliminating
Suicide-Related Behaviors

Identifying Behavioral Targets in Treatment:
Understanding the Suicidal Mode

Naturally, the distinguishing characteristics of the suicidal patient is the presence of suicidal thoughts and/or behaviors. Accordingly, this is one of the most prominent targets in treatment, particularly if treatment is time limited. This chapter discusses targeting the behavioral system of the suicidal mode including both suicide-related behaviors (i.e., suicidal acts and instrumental behaviors) and other possible self-destructive behaviors. Behavioral targets in the treatment of suicidality fall into three broad categories (see Figure 8.1):

1. Suicidal acts (i.e. suicide attempts with or without injuries).
2. Instrumental behaviors (with or without injuries).
3. Associated self-destructive behaviors (e.g., self-cutting/burning/piercing/hitting, substance abuse, risk taking behaviors [such as provoking others/fighting, driving fast or reckless, playing *Russian Roulette*], and promiscuity and unprotected sex, among a host of others).

For each suicide attempt, instrumental behavior, or episode of suicidality, the primary goal for the clinician is to articulate the *suicidal cycle*, that is, the sequence of thoughts, feelings, and behaviors that represent the suicidal mode *in action*. The clinician needs to target both obvious suicidality as well as re-

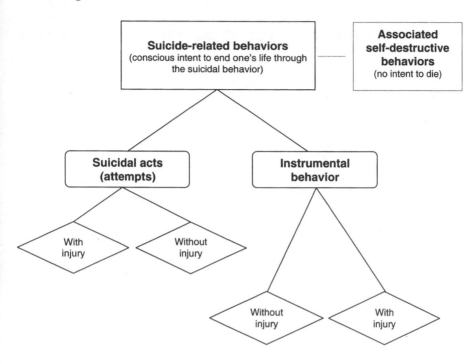

FIGURE 8.1. Conceptualizing the treatment of suicide-related behaviors.

lated problems with impulsivity and self-control. The opportunity exists to address both suicide-related behaviors as well as other self-destructive behaviors using the same conceptual model (see Figure 8.1). Consistent with the suicidal mode construct, the clinician will address cognitive, emotional, and behavioral aspects of suicide-related symptomatology (see Figure 8.2). A number of relatively broad questions provide the framework necessary to identify behavioral targets in treatment (see questions in Chapter 2 regarding outlining the suicidal mode).

Questions to Address Suicide-Related Behavior(s):

- What is the patient's history of suicidal behavior? How many attempts, what was the context for each, and what was the outcome (medically and psychologically)?
- What preparation, planning, or rehearsal behaviors has the patient engaged in?

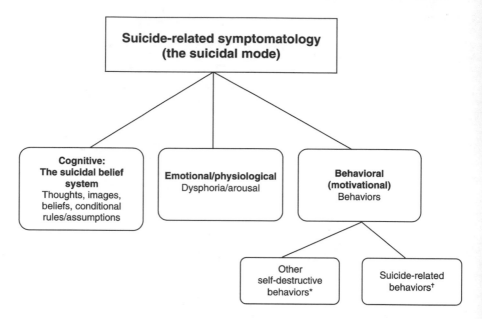

FIGURE 8.2. Conceptualizing suicide-related symptomatology using the suicidal mode. *No conscious intent to end one's life by suicide. Includes behaviors such as self-cutting/burning, piercing, substance abuse, risk-taking behaviors, and promiscuity, among others. †Conscious intent to end one's life by suicide. See Figure 6.1 for the distinction between suicidal acts and instrumental behavior.

- What is the patient doing to cope with his or her suicidality; that is, does the patient do anything to diffuse suicidal thinking right now (e.g., access his or her support system, isolate/withdraw, engage in substance abuse) or is the patient engaging in behaviors that only intensify the problem?
- What has the patient routinely done in response to past suicidal crises? Is there an identifiable pattern or trend to crises over time? Are the contextual variables (e.g., precipitant, response, and outcome) the same each time?

Questions to Address Impulsivity/Self-Control

- Is the patient evidencing impulsivity or problems with self-control? If so, in what manner (e.g., substance abuse, poor decision making, physical aggressiveness, and sexual acting out) and how frequently?
- Is impulsive behavior a characteristic feature of the patient's suicidality, regardless of intent?

- Have any impulsive behaviors resulted in injury or the need for medical care?
- What is the patient doing to regulate the prominent affect described during the crisis?
- How long does it take the patient to *recover* when acutely upset and dysphoric—a few second, minutes, hours, days?
- How long does it routinely take the patient to act on his or her thoughts during a crisis episode—a few seconds, a few minutes, hours, days?

Distinguishing between Suicidal Acts and Instrumental Behaviors

When outlining the suicidal mode and articulating the suicidal cycle for attempts and specific episodes of suicidality, it is critical to differentiate between suicidal acts and instrumental behaviors (see Figure 8.1). As evidenced in the nomenclature offered by O'Carroll et al. (1996), the distinguishing feature is intent. What did the patient intend to do? Did he or she want to die by suicide? Did the patient believe the method used was lethal? Did the patient take steps to prevent discovery? How was the patient discovered; was it by accident or unavoidable? How did the patient feel about surviving? If the intention was *not* death, what did the patient hope to accomplish? Distinguishing between subjective and objective intent also provides for a more thorough understanding of the patient's suicidal belief system. Specifically, it helps identify beliefs, conditional rules, and assumptions, as well as related compensatory strategies for the patient, all of which will be targeted directly. Most important, perhaps, it helps the clinician more clearly identify the patient's motivation for treatment and related risk status

As was discussed in Chapter 6, intent can frequently be difficult to gauge. A distinction was made between implicit (objective) intent and explicit (subjective) intent. When expressed or subjective intent matches with observed and reported behavior (implicit or objective intent), the treatment agenda is relatively straightforward. When the two conflict, an additional wrinkle is added to the treatment agenda—that is, the need to clarify the patient's intent and motivation for recovery and change. Specifically, identifying the intended purpose of the behavior is paramount. Articulating this purpose (e.g., emotion regulation, help seeking, and revenge) and helping the patient develop healthier and more effective skills quickly becomes the primary focus of treatment.

When outlining the suicidal cycle, it is important to clarify intent by addressing both subjective report and objective markers. In particular, it is important to focus on previous suicide attempts or specific episodes of suicidality. The patient's family members, a spouse, or significant others can also be of great assistance in clarifying any questions about the presence of instrumental behavior(s) and questionable intent. They frequently provide details that the patient might withhold and may well be able to provide evidence of habitual behavior not freely admitted. As was noted in Chapter 6, asking a series of clarifying questions such as the following can do this:

- "Did you think *taking an overdose* [i.e., statement of method] would kill you?"
- "What did you want to happen?"
- "Was medical care required? If so, what type and how did you access it?"
- "Did you get help after the suicide attempt?"
- "How were you discovered? Who discovered you?"
- "Did you take any steps to ensure that you wouldn't be discovered? If so, what steps did you take?"
- "Have you prepared for your suicide in any way? If so, what have you done?"
- "Have you rehearsed your suicide in any way [e.g., imagery versus actual behaviors]?"
- "How did you feel about surviving?"
- "What did you learn from your suicide attempt?

Prepatory behaviors consistent with implicit intent to suicide need to be routinely explored throughout the course of treatment but particularly during periods of acute crisis. Following are a series of entries from the diary of a patient who died by suicide, all indicative of methodical preparation and rehearsal that the patient purposefully withheld despite persistent and repetitive questioning. Although the patient withheld this information throughout a period of several months, it is important to note that on the day of his suicide he revealed it to his clinician. It was likely revealed only because of careful and persistent questioning such as that recommended. The circumstances of the patient's suicide were quite unusual. On the day of his suicide, he acknowledged the preparation referenced below and was promptly admitted to the hospital. On the way to the hospital in an ambulance, he assaulted one of the attendants, escaped, and later suicided after an extended and hostile standoff with police.

First entry

   "I bought a gun the other day. I didn't buy any ammo for some reason, but it's not too far off. I've been obsessed with my gun, thinking about it all the time."

Entry a few weeks later

"I fired my gun today; it's really loud. I fired five rounds. I've been seeing myself do it now, thinking about it, dreaming about it."

Entry a few months later

"I really flipped out today. I threw my ammo at someone in public. I almost lost it all. I know I have to do it now, because there is no help or relief for me now."

A few days after the final entry, the patient suicided using the gun described. A thorough and comprehensive review of the patient's prior and current suicide-related behaviors, with careful attention to clarifying intent, will it is hoped prevent such a tragic outcome. Far more often than not, intervention efforts are successful. Even in this tragic case, careful questioning ultimately revealed the patient's high-risk status and led to active efforts to have him hospitalized.

Dealing with Mixed Messages

Differences between the patient's expressed intent and his or her observed behavior (e.g., no expressed desire to die but repeated highly lethal attempts with injuries or high expressed intent and multiple, low-lethality attempts with certain discovery) can be the result of several and often multiple problems. Without question, a *mixed message* is a clear marker of problems and considerable ambivalence on the part of the patient. Each needs to be addressed directly in treatment and will likely hint at the need for longer-term care. Among the most frequent problems encountered are the following:

- Adequate rapport and a working therapeutic alliance have not been established. More time needs to be spent on developing a better therapeutic alliance (see Chapter 9), in all likelihood requiring time to be devoted to this issue each and every session.
- The patient's motivation for treatment is poor. The patient's commitment to the treatment process needs to be clarified, including expectations and responsibilities of both the patient and clinician (see later for more detailed discussion).
- The patient continues to be markedly ambivalent about suicide as an option. The patient needs to make a *commitment* to the treatment process. All that is being requested is that the patient agree to a *behavioral experiment*, simply experimenting to see if, after an identified period, he or she might *feel better*. The clinician simply need request that

the patient set aside suicide as an option for an identified period (e.g., 3 months, 6 months, or longer if necessary), while actively pursuing the treatment agenda.

- The patient's skill deficits prevent necessary interpersonal communication. If this is the case, the focus of treatment is on developing communication skills in order to establish the necessary working relationship and therapeutic alliance (see Chapter 9).
- The patient's symptoms are of adequate severity to impair cognitive functioning, motivation, and decision making. In such cases, symptom resolution is critical. Often this involves more intensive treatment (e.g., a partial hospital program, day treatment program, or hospitalization) as well as medication.
- The patient manifests significant personality psychopathology. In these cases, the patient's instrumental behaviors are made a central part of the treatment agenda, targeting the development of a healthier and more effective coping-skill repertoire.

Identifying the Suicidal Cycle

To understand the behavioral sequence, it is necessary to translate the suicidal mode into an episode-specific example—the suicidal cycle as discussed in Chapter 7. This is easiest to do with the patient's last episode of suicidality or, if the patient is actively suicidal, the current episode. As reviewed in Chapter 7, the clinician needs to work with the patient to identify the trigger(s), specific suicidal thoughts, associated feelings and physiological sensations, and ultimately behavioral outcomes (using the STR or simply strategic questioning). It is important to dissect the episode in as much detail as possible. As noted previously, careful questioning with respect to intent and outcome may lead to distinct behavioral targets critical to successful treatment. Implicit within the suicidal cycle is the treatment agenda, with each step representing a specific focus of intervention. A brief clinical example will help demonstrate this point further.

The Case of Mr. G (See Figure 8.3)

The patient was a middle-aged therapist who sought treatment after a protracted period of depression and the recent emergence of suicidal thoughts and what he described as a "near attempt." The patient reported that the near attempt occurred the previous week. He noted that he was returning home from work (trigger—the thought, feelings, or behavior associated with the onset of suicidality), started thinking that "things would never get any better" and decided "it would be better if he just killed himself" (fragmented

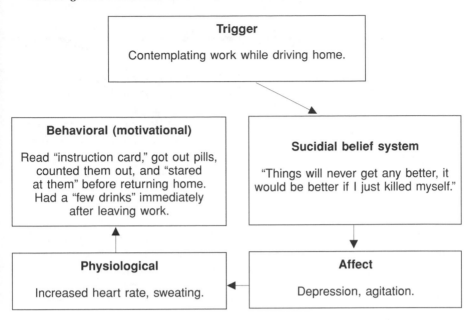

FIGURE 8.3. The suicidal cycle for Mr. G.

components of his suicidal belief system). He reported getting progressively more depressed and agitated as he drove for about the next 10–15 minutes (affect/physiological symptoms). When asked how he responded, the patient reported that he went to a bar, "had a few drinks" and ultimately "drove out to the lake" (behavior that exacerbates risk because it isolates him and alcohol consumption compounds the problem). He described sitting at the lake for some time and eventually stated that he "pulled out my instruction card and got the things necessary out of the trunk" (preparatory behavior). The patient had apparently written out "instructions" for his suicide on a 3 × 5 card that he kept in his wallet. The card, which was reviewed by the clinician, had a series of steps the patient needed to take "to successfully kill himself." He stated that he "wanted to make sure he didn't screw it up" when he was "emotional." He also had a "paper bag" with medications that he carried in the trunk of his car. He went on to describe "counting out his pills" (a preparatory behavior) and "staring at them for a long time" but eventually "packed things up" and returned home. He estimated that the entire episode lasted approximately 3 hours.

Depicting the suicidal cycle for Mr. G clearly articulates the treatment targets; that is, each step in the cycle represents a point for intervention (see Figure 8.3). It provides a more thorough understanding of the patient's potential risk and steps that need to be taken to reduce extreme or imminent risk. It helps make concrete what at times can be confusing for time-limited treatment.

Identifying the trigger can, at times, be somewhat complex. As is the case with Mr. G, it appears that his suicidal thoughts *just came out of nowhere.* However, closer scrutiny and discussion with Mr. G. revealed that it was the act of thinking about his day and his general dissatisfaction with work while driving home that triggered his suicidality. In other words, he *had time to stop and think* while driving home. Therefore, the trigger would be best described as *contemplating work while driving home.* This trigger revealed an underlying problem—the patient's long-standing dissatisfaction with his job and chosen profession.

Also of importance when depicting the suicidal cycle is to identify behaviors that only exacerbate suicide risk as well as those that might diminish risk. For Mr. G, isolating himself by driving out to the lake, consuming alcohol, and counting out his pills only exacerbate his risk. He had previously noted that he gets *more depressed* when alone and drinking. The availability of medication increases the likelihood of an impulsive overdose while he is intoxicated and dysphoric.

As evidenced for Mr. G, his particular suicidal cycle was of long duration, with no prominent impulsivity. It endured for an estimated 3 hours. Actually, Mr. G's methodical and compulsive planning are the hallmark features of his high-risk behavior. A careful review of his suicidal cycle revealed two important points for immediate intervention. First, Mr. G's access and availability to a plan and method needed to be promptly removed. This is consistent with one of the primary goals of crisis intervention reviewed in Chapter 7—always ensure the patient's safety. If he was adequately committed to treatment, an agreement needed to be reached in which he *gave up* his instruction card and stash of pills. In response, a more reasonable and healthier crisis response plan was developed and written down. Second, Mr. G's suicidal cycle revealed considerable time in which to implement a range of techniques to help him build skills and respond more effectively to his active suicidal belief system and acute emotional upset (see Chapter 9).

The Process of Behavioral Change: Reducing and Eliminating Suicidal Behavior

Reducing and, ultimately, eliminating suicide-related and other self-destructive behaviors in treatment requires that the following five steps be accomplished. Each step is then discussed in more detail, along with a few clinical examples.

1. The patient must make a commitment to treatment as an alternative to suicide. Without adequate commitment to the treatment process (e.g., attending sessions, setting goals, active involvement during sessions, openly voicing thoughts and feelings, and completing homework), little if any productive change will occur. Actually, without adequate commitment to change, treatment itself can inadvertently provide reinforcement and actually help maintain dysfunctional behavior(s).

2. The patient needs to develop an improved ability to self-monitor and better understand his or her particular suicidal cycle, with an emphasis on identifiable points for intervention and change.

3. There is a need to develop the ability (or skill) to inhibit the cycle. Initially, this will likely require late-cycle intervention (i.e., crisis intervention) but later will involve early-cycle intervention (i.e., skill building).

4. The patient will likely need to use simple substitute behaviors (i.e., short-term behavioral alternatives), if necessary, to alter or effectively inhibit the cycle.

5. The patient will need to develop and refine behavioral alternatives that are relatively permanent in nature. In an effort to permanently alter the suicidal cycle, the patient will need to respond to suicidal thoughts with behaviors that serve to diminish, rather than escalate, suicidality. This is, for the most part, consistent with a potentially substantial and enduring change in the patient's *way of living* or personality, with repetition and persistence of critical importance for those with chronic suicidality.

Making a Commitment to the Treatment Process

As with outcome in most psychotherapeutic approaches to a broad range of psychopathology, the patient's motivation for change and commitment to the treatment process are critical determinants of ultimate success (e.g., Roth & Fonagy, 1996). This is of particular importance in time-limited treatment. There is little time to waste, particularly if the patient presents with a relatively complex history, marked comorbidity (both Axis I and II), and chronic disturbance. An essential first step is to gain the patient's commitment to the treatment process. Although *ambivalence* is one of the most salient features of those presenting with suicidality (e.g., Shneidman, 1981, 1984, 1993), the ambivalence is clearly weighted in the direction of recovery given the simple fact that the patient is sitting in a clinician's office.

We recommend a relatively concrete and straightforward approach. Specifically, we encourage the use of a *commitment-to-treatment statement*, particularly for those manifesting chronic suicidality. As detailed in Figure 8.4, the statement essentially spells out the patient's responsibilities in treatment— that is, what the clinician expects the patient to do over both the short and long

I, _____ agree to make a commitment to the treatment process. I understand that this means that I have agreed to be actively involved in all aspects of treatment including:

1. Attending sessions (or letting my therapist know when I can't make it).
2. Setting goals.
3. Voicing my opinions, thoughts, and feelings honestly and openly with my therapist (whether they are negative or positive, but most importantly my negative feelings).
4. Being actively involved **during** sessions.
5. Completing homework assignments.
6. Experimenting with new behaviors and **new ways of doings things.**
7. Implementing my crisis response plan when needed.

I also understand and acknowledge that, to a large degree, a successful treatment outcome depends on the amount of energy and effort I make. If I feel like treatment is not working, I agree to discuss it with my therapist and attempt to come to a common understanding as to what the problems are and identify potential solutions. In short, **I agree to make a commitment to living.**

Signed:

_____

Date:

_____

Witness:

_____

FIGURE 8.4. Commitment to treatment statement. From *Treating Suicidal Behavior: An Effective, Time-Limited Approach* by M. David Rudd, Thomas Joiner, and M. Hasan Rajab. Copyright 2001 by The Guilford Press. Permission to reproduce this figure is granted to purchasers of this book for personal use only (see copyright page for details).

term. As is evident, we espouse a concrete approach to treatment in its entirety, consistently making the implicit *explicit*. As discussed in Chapter 9, this approach helps prevent the emergence or persistence of hidden agendas on the part of either the patient or clinician, resulting in a healthy and manageable *therapeutic belief system*.

Among the patient's responsibilities identified in Figure 8.4 are attending sessions; setting goals; voicing opinions, feelings, and thoughts in an open and honest manner; active involvement *during* sessions; experimenting with new behaviors and *new ways of doing things* outside sessions; completing homework assignments; and implementing the crisis response plan when necessary. As detailed in the statement, the patient is *making a commitment to living.* This approach is somewhat in contrast to traditional *no-suicide contracts* in that it does not detail what the patient *will not* do (i.e., suicide) but rather what he or she *will* do. We have found that suicidal patients, whether chronic or acute, are keenly aware of what they should not be doing but struggle to understand what other alternatives they have. Clearly articulating the patient's responsibilities from the outset helps establish a solid therapeutic relationship, enhancing the potential for a positive outcome.

The commitment-to-treatment statement should be presented as a part of the informed consent process. This is only one possible format for the statement. It can be modified and expanded, depending on the particular setting and clinical environment. Actually, the clinician and patient can simply sit down and draft their own statement in active collaboration. It is important to present the statement in a positive light, emphasizing the need to clearly articulate expectations and responsibilities, particularly given the theoretical importance of the suicidal mode and its cognitive component—the suicidal belief system. The rationale is fairly simply and should be conveyed to the patient as such. The more clear and specific we are throughout the entirety of the treatment process, the better the likelihood of success. The *statement* can be presented in the following manner:

> "Now that we've discussed your suicidal cycle and identified our initial treatment targets, I'd like to review the following statement with you. It articulates your commitment to the treatment process and identifies specific steps that you'll take in an effort to recover. In other words, it summarizes what's expected of you in treatment, your responsibilities. Although my responsibilities aren't summarized in the statement, we can spend a few minutes and discuss them now if needed. Why don't you review it [hands statement to the patient] and let me know your thoughts and feelings. Do you have any questions? Why don't we spend a few minutes and see if we can come to a working agreement?"

If the patient cannot, or does not, agree to the responsibilities outlined in the statement, issues of motivation for change and commitment to the treatment process need to be clarified and clearly articulated. Essentially, the clinician is are negotiating the treatment plan with the patient. It is hoped that he or she would be an active participant in the process. The presence of prominent ambivalence or hidden agendas will quickly surface if the patient balks at the statement. In all likelihood, this is a function of the patient's suicidal belief system. Chapter 9 discusses in detail approaches to targeting the suicidal belief system.

In addition to articulating the patient's responsibilities in treatment, it is important to discuss the clinician's responsibilities as well. In particular, it is important for the clinician to identify and discuss problems such as availability or accessibility, particularly during periods of acute crisis. Also, as discussed later, it is important for the clinician to be straightforward about what will occur if the patient fails to follow his or her crisis response plan (i.e., contingency management). If, for example, the clinician is never available on Fridays, it is important to point this out from the very beginning. If the setting in which the clinician works has a rotational call schedule, it needs to be clearly stated. A clear, definable set of expectations goes a long way to reducing problems later in treatment. This is particularly true if treatment is longer term. If expectations and responsibilities change during the course of treatment, this needs to be clarified. The commitment-to-treatment statement should be modified, amended, or simply rewritten and replaced if needed. Ideally all *statements* would be kept as a part of the permanent clinical record.

Making Sure the Patient Understands the Suicidal Cycle: Self-Monitoring and Emotional Awareness

For the most part, use of the STR and repetitive drawings of the suicidal cycle will improve the patient's ability to self-monitor, enhance his or her overall emotional awareness, and improve his or her general understanding of the suicidal cycle. Most important, though, self-monitoring provides a method to increase the amount of time available between the point at which the patient gets triggered and a suicide-related or self-destructive behavior emerges. As a result, there is more opportunity for intervention, experimentation with new behaviors, and ultimately productive skill building. The end result is an enhanced sense of personal control, power, and influence, all in stark contrast to prominent feelings of helplessness and hopelessness that characterized the patient's original presentation. In essence, the very act of self-monitoring provides a *behavioral experiment* to challenge core components of the suicidal belief system (see Chapter 9).

There are a broad range of self-monitoring tasks that can be used, including the STR, drawing the suicidal cycle, and the mood graph, all of which are described in Chapter 7. An hour-by-hour daily activity schedule (e.g., Hollon & Beck, 1979) can be used which provides considerable detail of day-to-day activities. This is sometimes helpful with patients who have a difficult time identifying specific triggering events. Along these lines, it is important to help the patient understand that triggering events can be internal (i.e., thoughts, images, feelings, or physical sensation) as well as external (situation or circumstance). An STR (or suicidal cycle) can subsequently be completed for each triggering event that is emotionally upsetting. Regardless of the method used, the primary goal of self-monitoring is to improve overall emotional awareness, creating opportunity for targeted intervention and behavioral change.

To transition from late- (i.e., crisis) to early-cycle intervention, self-monitoring will help the clinician identify *early markers* of suicidal crises. Early markers can include anything from specific thoughts (e.g., "I'd be better off dead") to feelings (e.g., severe anger or rage) to particular prepatory behaviors (e.g., reviewing will, organizing financial affairs, and letter writing). The important point is that if we can identify early markers, we can intervene with cognitive restructuring (Chapter 9), specific skills (Chapter 10), and substitute behaviors that diminish overall risk and, ultimately, suicide-related behaviors.

Inhibiting the Suicidal Cycle during Crisis States: Late-Cycle Intervention

Early in treatment, it is more likely that interventions will be late-cycle ones, consistent with crisis intervention discussed in Chapter 7. In other words, clinicians are likely to spend more time intervening *after* the patient is already suicidal. As discussed in detail in Chapter 7, *late-cycle interventions* revolve around a specific and detailed crisis response plan. The crisis response plan should include a step-by-step description of what the patient should do during a period of acute crisis. The plan should be modified as the patient's risk status, circumstances, and accessible skills change.

The goal for late-cycle interventions is simple—inhibit the emergence of a suicide-related or other self-destructive behavior. Late-cycle interventions are likely to rely on external support and the provision of direct clinical services (e.g., emergency sessions, telephone contacts, and consultation with other clinicians). Ideally, however, as treatment progresses late-cycle interventions would be managed entirely by the patient (i.e., consistent with the concept of symptom self-management and symptom utilization). If treatment were truly successful, the need for late-cycle interventions would eventually wane and disappear as suicidal crises become a thing of the past and the focus of treatment is addressing emotional upset, life stress, and daily hassles, all consistent with skill building.

The general guidelines for late-cycle interventions are fairly straightforward. They need to be *specific* (i.e., ideally written down step by step), *simple* (i.e. the patient should be able to complete the tasks during a state of acute emotional upset), and *accessible* (i.e., whatever the patient needs for the plan should be readily available, whether it is an exercise facility, a book, a stereo, or a particular person with whom to talk). For Mr. G, a possible late-cycle intervention is likely to be consistent with the crisis response plan detailed in Chapter 7.

> "*Crisis response plan:* When I'm upset and thinking about suicide, I'll take the following steps:
>
> "*Step 1.* Complete an STR and try to identify specifically what's upsetting me.
>
> "*Step 2.* Write out and review more reasonable responses to my suicidal thoughts, including thoughts about myself, others, and the future.
>
> "*Step 3.* Review all the conclusions I've come to about these thoughts in the past in my treatment log. For example, my job may be upsetting and I may get tired at times but in the past I have felt rejuvenated and more motivated if I simply take some time off. Although some aspects of the job have gotten more and more difficult, there are still things I love about it. In summary, I got into this job because I feel good about what I'm doing.
>
> "*Step 4.* Try to do the things that help me feel better for at least 30 minutes (listening to music, going to work out, reading my favorite novel, talking with my wife).
>
> "*Step 5.* Repeat all of the above.
>
> "*Step 6.* If the thoughts continue, get specific, and I find myself preparing to do something in an effort to make an attempt (e.g., taking out my pills and counting them), I'll call the emergency on-call person at XXX-XXXX.
>
> "*Step 7.* If I still feel suicidal and don't feel like I can control my behavior, I'll go to the emergency room. The phone number there is XXX-XXXX."

Substitute Behaviors and Purposeful Hypervigilance: Early-Cycle Intervention

As reliable *early markers* (i.e., prompts) of suicidal crises are clearly identified, the possibility of early-cycle intervention becomes more likely. For example, in the case of Mr. G, careful self-monitoring revealed that prior to his suicidal crises, a rather consistent pattern of behavior emerged. It was discovered that Mr. G would experience several days of escalating depression, consistent overeating of junk food, an abrupt halt of his exercise program, an emergence of thoughts such as "It's just not worth it," and gradual withdrawal and isolation from his family and support system. The end result was escalating depression and an emergence of suicidal thoughts.

To intervene effectively, the clinician and Mr. G identified a goal of *purposeful hypervigilance*. Specifically, Mr. G was to complete a daily activity schedule and watch (i.e., be purposefully hypervigilant) for the emergence of any of the *early markers* identified. When identified, Mr. G detailed on a coping card an early intervention plan which included the following steps (and formed the basis for a behavioral experiment as to whether or not this would make any difference in how he felt). Again, the plan needs to be simple, specific, and accessible. If the patient cannot readily implement the plan, then it is of no practical value when needed. It is important to be as specific and detailed as possible, even putting dates and times when appropriate.

"Early intervention plan

"1. Ensure that, during periods of significant stress, time (at least 30 minutes) is made to eat three meals a day. Limit snacking on junk food. Try to eliminate it entirely during the workday.
"2. Implement an exercise plan that includes exercising at the gym on Monday, Wednesday, and Friday for an hour on each occasion, preferably from 7:00 to 8:00 P.M.
"3. Make sure that at least 8 hours per day is set aside for sleep, in bed by 11 P.M. and up at 7 A.M.
"4. Complete a daily STR targeting any morbid or suicidal thoughts. I can set aside time at the end of lunch every day given that it will only take about 5 minutes or so.
"5. Access support system on a regular basis. Make sure to spend time with children each and every day. Also, attend church on a weekly basis and make time for *a date* with my wife, possibly every 2 to 3 weeks. This will mean having to get a regular babysitter, something my wife has agreed to coordinate."

As evidenced in the example provided, early intervention plans need to be specific (preferably written) and tied to specific early markers of suicidality. In addition, the early intervention plan can be framed as a behavioral experiment, essentially testing an identifiable component of the patient's suicidal belief system (e.g., "Nothing will help me feel better"; see Chapter 8 for a detailed discussion). Furthermore, all patients should be encouraged to summarize any resultant conclusions in their treatment log or journal.

Shaping Behavior: A Process of Gradual Change

For the most part, the process described in this chapter is generally consistent with the concept of behavior *shaping* and *contingency management* (e.g., Craighead, Craighead, Kazdin, & Mahoney, 1994). Shaping refers to the process of reinforcing relatively small steps or approximations of a targeted, desired behavior (e.g., assertiveness, effective anger management, and problem solving). This is often necessary in treating suicidal behavior. Contingency management is rooted in operant learning principles and refers to the process of reinforcing positive behaviors, whereas negative behaviors are met with either a neutral or negative consequence. The therapeutic relationship and the treatment environment itself need to be structured in such a way as to allow for effective contingency management (see later).

Suicide-related and other self-destructive behaviors are the result of a complex web of factors, particularly for those with chronic suicidality. A series of small steps will, in all likelihood, be necessary to initially reduce and ultimately eliminate the suicidal response. For the majority of patients, this requires late-cycle intervention using the crisis response plan, modifying it as needed or indicated by the patient's observed progress. Early-cycle intervention will follow, consisting primarily of behavioral experiments and skill acquisition and refinement exercises, all of which have a considerable influence on the structural content of the patient's suicidal belief system.

For those evidencing instrumental behavior(s), it is important to consistently explore the purpose or intent of the behavior and evaluate its overall effectiveness at achieving the end goal, as well as ultimately, its negative consequences. In particular, those manifesting instrumental behaviors will consistently recognize three things about their behavior. First, it in all likelihood did not accomplish the goal intended. Second, it had negative interpersonal consequences, probably damaging (if not ending) an existing relationship in some form or fashion. And, third, it resulted in considerable self-image damage, reinforcing negative self-image beliefs that have persisted for years and serve as the foundation of the suicidal belief system.

For those evidencing instrumental behaviors, a solid therapeutic relationship is critical. The therapeutic relationship can be used as a vehicle for change, consistently addressing and evaluating the three conclusions summarized earlier. For each episode involving instrumental behavior, the clinician needs to ask three relatively simple questions and be persistent in reinforcing the conclusions drawn:

> [after having completed a suicidal cycle for an episode several days ago] "Let's take a look at what happened last week. Did you accomplish what you had hoped to? You said you wanted to get back at Jim [boyfriend] for what he did? Did that actually happen?" [failure to accomplish stated goal]

[a few minutes later] "Rather than hurt Jim in some way, it sounds like you actually ended up in a fight with your mother? Actually, from what you said, it sounded like you hurt your mother's feelings? Does this sound accurate?" [negative interpersonal consequence]

[still later in the session] "From what you describe, it sounds as though you had some very negative thoughts about yourself. You also mentioned feeling very guilty. Do you recall some of the beliefs you've held about yourself over time [inadequacy, worthlessness, incompetence, unlovable]? In some ways, it sounds like what happened only served to reinforce these ideas? What do you think, does this sound accurate?" [reinforcement of negative self-image and components of the patient's suicidal belief system]

Exposure-Based Strategies: Role Playing, Cue Exposure, and Behavioral Rehearsal

As discussed in more detail in Chapter 10, a number of exposure-based strategies are helpful to ensure the effectiveness of early- and late-cycle intervention efforts. Role playing (and role reversal) is particularly effective if the crisis response or intervention plan includes interpersonal issues, which it almost always does. What essentially amounts to cue exposure or targeted behavioral (i.e., repeated exposure to a particularly troubling cue or prompt in order to facilitate not only desensitization in terms of the emotional response but adequate coping behaviors) is helpful when there is marked emotional upset and impulsivity (e.g., self-cutting/burning/piercing in response to perceived rejection). Behavioral rehearsal is universally helpful, allowing the patient an opportunity to simply rehearse the crisis response or early-intervention plan repetitively (through imagery or individual repetition or through role playing if the issue is interpersonal in nature). The usefulness of each of these techniques can be enhanced by videotaping and regular review and discussion of the tapes. Chapter 10 discusses each of these techniques in considerable detail.

Contingency Management and Treatment Success

As a part of the initial informed consent process and review of the commitment-to-treatment statement, it is important to articulate the contingency management strategy that will be used in treatment, in other words, the limits and boundaries that will characterize the treatment relationship. This needs to be done as early as reasonably possible. Such articulation is of particular importance for those who evidence chronic suicidality and make multiple attempts. Essentially, the question that needs to be answered is, What will you do when the patient does not follow his or her crisis response or early-intervention plan?

In these cases, the therapeutic relationship itself can be used quite effectively if the clinician has clearly articulated the limits and boundaries of the relationship. Contingency management is most appropriate, and effective, in response to emergency presentations. Limiting phone calls, emergency sessions, or follow-up sessions can be used as a judicious, natural negative consequence for those with chronic suicidality who fail to follow their identified plans. For example, if a patient did not follow the crisis response plan and is subsequently hospitalized, it would be appropriate for the clinician to limit individual sessions for a while (while the patient adjusts to the inpatient unit), and potentially until discharge. This is consistent with establishing clear limits and boundaries for the patient when articulating the treatment plan—and sticking to them throughout the duration of treatment. If a patient abuses telephone calls, it would be appropriate to limit phone calls (e.g., one per week initially), eventually tapering them down. If the abuse is severe, deferring calls to the emergency coverage team *on call* would be appropriate. Regardless of the contingency management strategies used, it is important to clearly articulate them and discuss them early in the treatment process. Although all clinical settings have unique characteristics, we recommend a few general guidelines about contingency management:

- Clearly articulate crisis availability and accessibility. This is of particular importance for those patients with chronic suicidality. Regardless of the clinician's own availability, 24-hour emergency services need to be available to the patient in some form or fashion. Will the clinician return telephone calls? If so, within what time frame. What is the clinician's availability for emergency or *work-in* sessions? How frequently? Under what conditions? If the clinician not a part of a rotational call roster, he or she must let the patient know.
- Clearly articulate the definition of crisis for the patient. This should be done as a part of the *crisis response plan* illustrated earlier and in Chapter 6. Implicit within the plan are specific conditions under which to access emergency services.
- Clearly define availability and accessibility for between-session contact when the patient is *not* in crisis. For example, the patient might want to contact the clinician to clarify a point about a treatment goal or a specific behavioral experiment. This is perhaps the most effective way to reinforce productive change and healthy behaviors. This can be made a standard part of the patient's *early-intervention plan*. If the patient gets *stuck* at some point during early intervention, a phone call for clarification, motivation, and support can be tremendously effective.
- Minimize the need for external intervention or support (i.e., from the

clinician) as much as is possible, all the while recognizing that early in treatment external support may be essential. This is consistent with the idea of symptom self-management and symptom utilization. The primary goal is to help the patient to develop the skills necessary to manage and respond to crises effectively and independently.

• Consistently reinforce independent functioning and the emergence of new behavioral responses that, frequently, the patient might not be fully aware of. This is relatively easy to do during session. For example, the clinician can routinely say, "It sounds like you've again accomplished one of your primary goals, that is, to handle crises on your own and in an effective manner." The clinician can go a step further and also address specific implications for the patient's suicidal belief system by adding, "What does this say about your ability, your competency and some of the other things you've believed about yourself over the years? What conclusions could you come to about your skills?"

Naturally, reinforcement of appropriate behaviors is a focus throughout the entirety of treatment. Of particular importance is reinforcement of the patient's independent functioning. This is accomplished each and every session. Having patients draw conclusions about their previously identified suicidal belief system and record them in their treatment log is particularly effective (see Chapter 8). Regardless, consistent and persistent reinforcement of independent functioning is critical. Careful and comprehensive thinking about contingency management before treatment begins ensures that this will happen.

Targeting Treatment Disruptions

A number of additional steps can be taken to facilitate openness and overall responsiveness of the patient throughout the course of treatment. What have been traditionally referred to as transference–countertransference reactions, as well as patient resistance and provocations, are all discussed in more detail in the next section. A broader construct, *treatment disruptions*, need to be addressed from the very first session. Early therapeutic interactions will, in many ways, determine success later on in the process. Each time the clinician addresses a problem that disrupts the treatment process, he or she is establishing the ground rules for therapy, even if implicit rather than explicit. As has been stated earlier, it is important to make the implicit explicit and talk clearly and concretely about problems. Treatment disruptions include anything that *disrupts the ability to conduct outpatient treatment in a predictable, consistent, reliable, and productive manner.* The most frequent problems surface around issues of session attendance and duration, recurrent crises, and difficulty adhering to the treatment agenda. Among examples are the following:

- Frequently missed appointments.
- Rescheduled appointments.
- Brief appointments.
- Appointments of inordinate length (e.g., a couple of hours).
- An inordinate number of phone calls.
- Recurrent crises that distract from continuity in the treatment agenda.
- The need for frequent consultations (i.e. psychiatric and otherwise) and recurrent evaluations for hospitalization.
- Frequent hospitalizations.
- Persistent hostility and anger directed at the clinician.
- Failure to complete homework assignments.

We recommend that the clinician keep track of treatment disruptions as a part of the routine clinical entry, noting the frequency and severity of the problem, whether or not it was discussed, and the nature of the subsequent response. Treatment disruptions can be discussed directly with the patient in a nonthreatening, empathetic manner. Addressing such disruptions directly, as needed, not only facilitates resolution of the problem for more efficient and effective treatment but models a healthy and functional relationship for the patient. To address these issues in a nonthreatening manner, a relatively methodical approach can be followed:

1. State the problem clearly, making it a treatment issue, not a problem with the patient individually.
2. Frame it within the context of the patient's current emotional pain, that is, that it is a function of the very problems that brought the patient to treatment.
3. Request any needed clarification from the patient until both patient and clinician agree with respect to the specific problem (i.e., maintain an alliance).
4. Offer a specific solution.
5. Request any needed clarification from the patient until both patient and clinician agree with respect to the solution.
6. Reinforce the patient's ability to identify, discuss, and resolve the problem.

For example:

THERAPIST: I was wondering if you noticed that our last three sessions have all run about twenty minutes over [a specific problem, not attributed specifically to the patient]? I think part of the reason is that we've been addressing some recent problems that have been fairly urgent and quite upsetting to you [provided context]? Additionally, some of these things haven't come up until the end of the session(s). Would you agree or am I off the mark a little here [clarification]?

PATIENT: Yeah, I think you're right. I've felt like I haven't had enough time and you seem rushed. I've really gotten mad at you about it [willingness to discuss the therapeutic relationship].

THERAPIST: It sounds like maybe the problem is that we haven't had enough time given some of the things going on in your life right now [clarification].

PATIENT: I think that's right, I'd like more time.

THERAPIST: Perhaps we should meet twice a week for the next three weeks until some of the current problems are dealt with a little more effectively [specific solution]?

PATIENT: I'd like that [agreement].

THERAPIST: OK, let's get with my secretary to set that up. I just wanted to point out how effectively you're discussing problems, regardless of what they are, and coming up with solutions. What we just talked about is only one example [reinforcement]. I'll remind you that exactly one of the things we established as a goal when you first started. Also, as we've discussed before, many of the interpersonal problems you've struggled with, such as expressing anger, would come up in the therapy relationship. I just want to say that you've handled it very well.

The following section emphasizes the effective management of hostility and provocations, described by Newman (1997) as client emotional abuse, in treatment. Given that the model provided here is consistent with CBT, an alternative approach to the traditional psychoanalytic constructs of transference–countertransference is needed. Traditional psychodynamic constructs simply do not fit very well. They are theoretically and conceptually incongruous.

Provocation(s): The Currency of Interpersonal Relatedness in Suicidality

Any clinician working with suicidal patients for any amount of time quickly comes to recognize that provocations are part and parcel of psychotherapy for suicidality. In short, they should be expected. It is incumbent on the clinician to manage provocations in a caring, sensitive, patient, professional, and effective fashion. This is the battlefield in which trust, fortitude, patience, and compassion will all be severely tested. For some patients, this is not an issue. For others, such as those with chronic suicidality, it is often a *rite of passage* that frequently is unavoidable, despite our best efforts. It can be, however, managed efficiently and effectively. Clearly, though, this is easier said than done. To effectively deal with severe provocations during the course of treatment, the clinician will have to possess a high tolerance for criticism, be confident in his or her clinical skills, exhibit considerable patience, and think clearly and effectively when pressured. Also, social support and access to clinical consultation are paramount. Every clinician needs to persistently remind him- or herself that this is simply one of the problems with which the patient is struggling and guard against personalizing provocations in any manner. As stated earlier, the mantra of *expect it* (understand it), *prepare for it, and resolve it* applies.

As Maltsberger and Buie (1974, 1989) have eloquently described, the provocative behavior of the chronically suicidal patient can be unrelenting. They have defined and described three categories of provocations (see Table 8.1):

1. Direct verbal devaluations of the therapist. For example: "You really don't know what you're doing, I'd be better off seeing my friend for therapy, at least they don't say things that screw me up! I might as well just kill myself now and get this over with!"
2. Direct actions or behaviors including tantrums, inconvenient phone calls, missed appointments, general acting out such as coming to sessions intoxicated, letter writing, drawings, or recurrent attempts of low lethality.
3. Indirect actions or behaviors such as silence or refusal to talk during sessions, general noncompliance or arguing over trivialities during sessions, nonspecific repeated somatic complaints, "forgetting."

TABLE 8.1. Classification of Provocations and Examples

Category	Examples
Direct	*Verbal devaluations:* "You really don't know what you're doing. You're incompetent, how'd you ever get a license. This will never work. I might as well kill myself now." *Direct actions or behaviors:* Tantrums, repeated phone calls, missed appointments, repeatedly being late for appointments, frequent cancellations, intoxication, letter writings, drawings, recurrent attempts of low lethality (with no intent).
Indirect	*Indirect actions or behaviors:* Silence, refusal to talk, general noncompliance, arguing of trivial issues, non-specific somatic complaints (e.g., muscle pain, hurting all over), forgetting to complete homework, forgetting what was addressed last session, forgetting identified goals or targets.

Similarly, Newman (1997) has defined client emotional abuse as "a pattern of hostile, undercontrolled, or otherwise emotionally provocative verbal behavior and boundary infringements that are directed at the therapist and are not readily diminished by the therapist's appropriate actions" (p. 4). In addition, Newman (1997) cautions that persistent abusive behavior represents "an ongoing misuse of the therapeutic relationship" (p. 5), providing an opportunity for the patient to express potentially sadistic motivations and to not use the therapeutic relationship in a meaningful manner, failing to identify and experiment with new and more effective interpersonal skills. He goes on to offer specific recommendations for the management of client emotional abuse, including cognitive and imaginal rehearsal; rationally responding to excessive self-reproach and angry ruminations; use of flashcards, mottos, and "all purpose self-statements"; consultation and social support; development of communication skills and assertiveness; and appropriate assertive communication in session. In terms of assertive communication in session, Newman (1997) recommends the following steps:

1. Change accusations into requests.
2. Demonstrate respect for yourself and the client.
3. Reflect before retorting.
4. Never use profanity or insulting epithets.
5. Avoid cognitive distortions in your communication (e.g., "This always . . . ").
6. Use *we* statements.

Newman summarizes his recommendations with the following: "Do not abandon your standard clinical policies in an attempt to mollify an emotionally abusive, undercontrolled client; instead, politely give the rationale for maintaining your position, and document the interaction in your notes, emphasizing the cost-benefit analysis involved in choosing one intervention over the other" (p. 21).

In the treatment of suicidality, provocations can take many forms. As summarized by Maltsberger and Buie (1974, 1989) they can manifest either directly or indirectly. They can cover the full gamut of suicidal behaviors, from potentially lethal to low-lethality attempts. The critical issue is the motivation or intent of the behavior (as reviewed in Chapter 6). If the intent was something other than death (e.g., emotional relief, anger expression, revenge, or punishment of another), the behavior can be conceptualized as potentially provocative. For example, a female patient said that she was going to go to home, get a razor, come back and cut her wrist if one of the authors refused to hold her hand in session as her last therapist did. Provocations can come in the form of letters, drawings, poems, or audiotapes. The defining characteristic of provocative communication is that it is an expression of extreme emotional upset or dysphoria (e.g., anger, fatigue, and frustration) that is intended to elicit a response from the therapist.

The salience and significance of provocation in the treatment of suicidality should be apparent. In a sense, every provocation is an opportunity to solidify the therapeutic relationship, enhance the treatment agenda, and advance patient growth and development. It is important to weave the management of provocations into the treatment process, identifying provocations as simply another skill deficit to be addressed. However, it is critical to recognize that in effectively addressing provocations, we must not reinforce them, covertly or overtly.

Handling Provocation in Treatment

We recommend a three-step approach to managing provocations. The three steps include (1) exploring the patient's feelings, (2) helping the patient understand the basic patterns of provocative communication, and (3) introducing the patient to alternative ways to solve interpersonal problems (see Figure 8.5). Of primary importance is not to reinforce provocations in any fashion, covertly or overtly. As is apparent, intermittent reinforcement is perhaps the most powerful means to shape a behavior, so consistency is vital.

Strategies for Step 1: Exploring the Patient's Feelings

1. Attend to, label, and reflect the patient's feelings (e.g., anger, frustration, and irritation) in a nonjudgmental, nondefensive fashion. For example: "You sound very upset and angry with me about the appointment that had to be canceled."

2. Elicit any additional thoughts or feelings about the therapist, the treatment process, or the patient's current situation. In other words, define the current context for the provocation. For example: "Is that on target or would you like to add to that? How are you feeling about your treatment, do you have any concerns about how things are going in general? I realize that things have been very stressful lately."

3. Reinforce the appropriate expression of negative affect or, if the expression was inappropriate (e.g., a tantrum), place the problem within the treatment context. For example: "I just want to let you know that is good to see you bring difficult feelings and problem up in such an appropriate way." Or (if a tantrum), "You may not have brought this up in the way you'd hoped, but this is something we need to work on, something you'd identified as a prob-

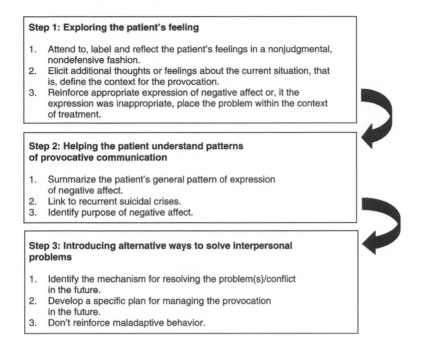

Step 1: Exploring the patient's feeling

1. Attend to, label and reflect the patient's feelings in a nonjudgmental, nondefensive fashion.
2. Elicit additional thoughts or feelings about the current situation, that is, define the context for the provocation.
3. Reinforce appropriate expression of negative affect or, it the expression was inappropriate, place the problem within the context of treatment.

Step 2: Helping the patient understand patterns of provocative communication

1. Summarize the patient's general pattern of expression of negative affect.
2. Link to recurrent suicidal crises.
3. Identify purpose of negative affect.

Step 3: Introducing alternative ways to solve interpersonal problems

1. Identify the mechanism for resolving the problem(s)/conflict in the future.
2. Develop a specific plan for managing the provocation in the future.
3. Don't reinforce maladaptive behavior.

FIGURE 8.5. A stepwise approach to responding to provocations.

lem for years, that is, your ability to tell someone that your mad in a way you can feel good about or proud of."

Strategies for Step 2: Helping the Patient Understand the Basic Patterns of Provocative Communication

1. Summarize the patient's general pattern of expression of negative affect. For example: "As we've discussed from time to time, and as you've noted from the beginning, one of the problems that you've run into is expressing anger in a direct manner so we can discuss it openly and solve whatever the problem is."

2. Link to recurrent suicidal crises. For example: "As we discussed when we put the model down on paper, you mentioned that you end up feeling really down and guilty when your anger comes out this way, and a lot of the time you ended up wanting to kill yourself to get rid of the feeling."

3. Identify the purpose of the negative affect. For example: "After talking about this a little more, it sounds like what you really wanted was to just

let me know that you were not pleased about the appointment that had been cancelled. Is that accurate?"

Strategies for Step 3: Introducing Alternative Ways to Solve Interpersonal Problems

1. Identify the mechanism for resolving the problems/conflicts in the future. For example: "Let me suggest that if you feel this way in the future that we make it an item on the agenda for the session, maybe the first thing we talk about. Or if you'd like to address it differently, just let me know. Do you have any ideas about how we might address this?"

2. Develop a specific plan for managing the provocation in the future. For example: "How would you feel about discussing a plan for handling anger in the future? For example, you might want to write about it in your journal, use your daily thought record, audiotape your thoughts and feelings, or write me a letter if needed. Then, after you've clarified the problem, you can just put it on the session agenda and we'll pursue it like we do every other goal."

It is important to develop strategies in handling provocations that do not reinforce maladaptive coping or self-destructive behaviors. The response should be measured and strategically target the patient's specific situation, naturally depending on assessed risk. For example, a patient stormed out the office near the end of a session in response to the clinician's comment about a potential benefit of his brooding withdrawal and self-imposed isolation:

PATIENT: I got really mad at her [wife], so I just stayed in the bedroom all day, didn't say a thing to her.

THERAPIST: Did she know you were angry or why?

PATIENT: Oh, she got the message.

THERAPIST: How so?

PATIENT: Every time she came in the room I gave her "that" look. After a couple of hours she came in and apologized and was really nice.

THERAPIST: It sounds like that, in a way, you got what you wanted, did you feel good about the way it happened?

PATIENT: Screw you. . . . (*Storms out of room.*)

In the case summarized, the clinician chose not to go after the patient. That is, not to reinforce his behavior. The patient was not actively suicidal, had been stabilized for some time, and had made nice progress in treatment and a good working alliance was in place. Rather than going after him, the clinician decided to call the next day to ensure the patient was doing well (i.e., maintain the alliance) and, using the steps summarized earlier, denote that the problem was recurrent in nature and one the patient ultimately felt badly about. After a brief discussion, the patient agreed and it was placed on the agenda for the next session.

The Evolution of Hope and the Elimination of Suicidal Behavior: A Few Concluding Words

Without doubt, as the patient feels more hopeful about the future, suicidality will diminish. However, it is important to note that for many chronic patients, this will require the development and refinement of skills that have long been dormant or simply absent. In these cases, time will be a critical determinant of treatment success. At the heart of the issue, regardless, is a strong therapeutic relationship and alliance. Even when under considerable stress and when the patient has hope about little else, it is important that the therapeutic relationship be a predictable, dependable, reliable resource. It needs to be a resource about which there is little confusion; a resource that clearly states the ground rules and does not have hidden agendas and competing needs. In other words, it needs to be entirely different from many of the patient's other relationships. In many cases, hope is often a function of predictability. It is not a bad thing to hear from a patient something like, "I knew you'd say that." It is not enough to simply know that the clinician will *be there*. It is important for the patient to know what the clinician will do and how he or she will respond, regardless of the circumstance. This is accomplished by clearly articulating expectations and responsibilities regarding the treatment process, along with the use of an effective contingency management strategy.

9

Cognitive Restructuring:
Changing the Suicidal Belief
System and Building a Philosophy
for Living

This chapter focuses specifically on cognitive restructuring, that is, modifying the structure and content of the suicidal mode and related facilitating modes. Chapter 9 addresses the issue of skill building, consistent with the idea of *constructing more adaptive modes* in an effort to ensure productive and lasting change. Many of the techniques reviewed here are consistent with those used in traditional cognitive therapy (e.g., Beck, 1964, 1976; Beck, Freeman, & Associates, 1990; J. S. Beck, 1995), representing what has become a relatively common trend in cognitive therapy—a problem-specific variation and adaptation.

Private Meaning and the Suicidal Belief System: The Role of Automatic Thoughts and Intermediate and Core Beliefs

Many of the clinical techniques developed in cognitive therapy over the years have been well tested and applied quite effectively to a broad range of clinical problems such as major depression, generalized anxiety, panic, social phobia, substance abuse, and personality disorders (e.g., Arnkoff & Glass, 1992; Hollon & Beck, 1993, for reviews). Although the techniques employed have been similar, each has varied in accordance with the unique characteristics of the particular problem(s) being targeted. Despite variations, there has been one identifiable consistency in the approaches referenced; the central pathway for the psychopathology targeted has been conceptualized as cognition, the *private* meaning assigned by the individual.

In cognitive therapy, *private* meaning is apparent in the patient's automatic thoughts, intermediate beliefs, and underlying core beliefs. With respect to the suicidal belief system, automatic thoughts are a "manifest stream of thinking that coexists with an underlying stream of thought such as a core belief" (J. S. Beck, 1995, pp. 10–11), intermediate beliefs are basically rules and assumptions for daily living, and core beliefs comprise the actual content of the schemas and are the product of the individual's developmental history. As illustrated in Figure 9.1, there is a hierarchical relationship between the three, with automatic thoughts providing a clue that a core belief of the suicidal belief system is active, along with related conditional rules and assumptions. As illustrated with the case of Mr. G, when a patient is suicidal, core beliefs are active in three distinct areas, including self, others, and the future. Naturally, the three are interrelated, tied together by the thread of hopelessness (i.e., the belief that the situation or *life circumstance* will not change appreciably, at least not enough to *go on living*). The hierarchy illustrated in Figure 9.1 is

---

Automatic thoughts: During the active suicidal belief system
Self (unlovable): "I'm a loser, I should die, I should kill myself."
Other (rejecting): "Bob hates me."
Future (hopeless): "It's hopeless."

Intermediate beliefs: Rules and assumptions
"If I do everything right, if I'm perfect, then people will accept me." **(perfectionism)**
"If I'm perfect then I'll deserve to live." **(perfectionism)**
"If I do what others want then they'll accept me." **(subjugation)**

Core beliefs: The suicidal belief system
Self (unlovable): "I'm worthless, I don't deserve to live."
Others (rejecting): "Nobody really cares about me."
Future (hopeless): "Things will never change."

FIGURE 9.1. The relationship between active core beliefs of the suicidal belief system, intermediate beliefs, and automatic thoughts: The case of Mr. G.

simply a more detailed outline of the cognitive system of the suicidal mode. That is, it represents the observable or manifest content of a negative core belief underlying the patient's intent (desire) to die by suicide.

Beck (1995) described a number of characteristics of automatic thoughts including that they tend to be *relatively brief*, are often *shorthand* for a more detailed belief, and can be in imagery form rather than verbal form. Intermediate beliefs are, for the most part, the patient's rules and assumptions for daily living. They represent a translation of the patient's compensatory strategies (e.g., perfectionism, subjugation, avoidance, and withdrawal) into verbal, descriptive form. For example, in the case of Mr. G, perfectionism (i.e., one of his primary compensatory strategies) manifests as "if I'm perfect then I deserve to live." Core beliefs, and negative core beliefs specifically, tend to be absolute in quality and pervasive in impact, corrupting individual perception. Beck (1995) hypothesized two categories of core beliefs, those associated with *helplessness* and those associated with *unlovability*. She went on to note that all negative core beliefs can, in some form or fashion, be categorized within one of these two broad factors. For suicidal patients, frequently, core beliefs are active in both domains. As with Mr. G, not only does he feel *worthless* (unlovability), but he expresses an inability to change his situation to any substantial degree (helplessness). In addition, however, it is important to remember that the patient's suicidal belief system involves core beliefs about *others* as well as about the future. Future beliefs are, naturally, characterized as hopeless. Beliefs about *others* are most frequently characterized as *rejecting* in some fashion (e.g., rejecting, abandoning, abusing, critical, and judgmental). Core beliefs in all three areas, the entirety of the cognitive triad (i.e., self, others, future), need to be targeted in order to effectively restructure the suicidal belief system.

Identifying automatic thoughts, conditional rules and assumptions (i.e., intermediate beliefs), and core beliefs (across all three areas of the cognitive triad) is fairly straightforward with the suicidal patient. Consistent with the acute overlay to the suicidal presentation, the suicidal belief system is active and accessible during session(s). The STR is a readily accessible source from which to detail the suicidal belief system but can be quickly expanded by asking a few critical questions:

- What are the patient's reasons for dying (self-component of the cognitive triad)? Why does he or she want to die right now? For example, "I'm worthless, I can't do anything right" (unlovability); "I'm going to kill myself because my wife is divorcing me; I'm a loser" (unlovability); "I can't live without her; I can't stand feeling this way anymore" (helplessness); "I'll never be able to get another job" (helplessness).

- How does the patient describe him- or herself (self-component of the cognitive triad) when actively suicidal? "I'm inadequate and incompetent, that's why I got fired" (unlovability); "I'm so ashamed of the things I've done; I don't deserve to go on living" (unlovability); "I'm a murderer; I deserve to die" (unlovability).
- How does the patient describe others? What is the nature and quality of current relationships (other-component of cognitive triad)? "I'll never have a good relationship, everybody I've ever dated left" (rejecting, abandoning). "All she ever did was criticize me, tell me what a terrible person I was" (rejecting, critical, and judgmental).
- What must happen in order for him or her to feel better (conditional rules/assumptions, compensatory strategies)? "If I could just do everything right, then I'd be OK" (perfectionism). "If I just do what people want me to, then they'll accept me" (subjugation). "If I just stay to myself and get lost for a while, maybe things will get better or this will all go away" (avoidance, withdrawal).

Given the circumstances unique to suicidality, seldom will the suicidal belief system be inactive when the patient is present for treatment. Occasionally, however, with a chronically suicidal patient, the suicide belief system may be difficult to access during periods of relative stability and calm (even if short-lived). The questions noted previously will, in all likelihood, unearth the suicide belief system. However, the clinician can also *activate the suicide belief system* by having the patient focus on the most recent episode of suicidality. The following steps are recommended:

1. Have the patient describe the last attempt or episode in detail, both with respect to precipitant(s), the attempt or episode itself (i.e., *what* was done, *when* it was done, and under what *circumstances*), and outcome (i.e., medically and psychologically). Essentially, complete the suicidal cycle described earlier in Chapters 6 and 7 that is necessary to illustrate the suicidal mode in action. For example, the patient might describe the following:

"I can remember right after he broke up with me. I started thinking about killing myself, that I couldn't go on without him. We had been together for five years; I couldn't see my life without him in it. That first night, it was about 1 A.M., I went and got all my medication. I counted out the pills. I drank three, maybe four, beers and just looked at the pills. Then I got out a sheet of paper and wrote a note to him and my parents. I took all of the pills and lay down on the couch. I listened to the radio for a while and then started to get really groggy. I got scared and called my mom. I don't remember anything from there. I woke up in the ER sometime later. I think they had pumped by stomach and made me drink this 'charcoal stuff.' At the time, I was really disappointed to wake up. It's weird, isn't it? I wanted to die, got scared, and then was disappointed that I lived."

2. Focus on and describe all components of the suicidal mode, including thoughts, feelings, related physical sensations, and associated behaviors. "Do you remember how you felt right after he broke up with you? Are you having any of those feelings right now? How'd you feel after taking the pills? You said you got scared and then later you mentioned being disappointed? What did you feel physically earlier in the night, how about later?"

3. Once evidence of a marked *affect shift* is observed, revisit the questions listed earlier. Any observed negative *affect shift* is evidence that the suicidal mode has been activated.

Consistent with the idea of ensuring adequate structure and organization to time-limited work, it is helpful to organize the patient's beliefs about self and others so that they can be more efficiently and effectively targeted in treatment. Beliefs about the future are almost always uniformly hopeless during periods of acute suicidality and not a particular concern. Beliefs about self and others can be organized in a relatively simple fashion by having the patient keep a *running hierarchy* of identified beliefs in his or her treatment log (see Figure 9.2). As is apparent in Figure 9.2, the beliefs listed are fairly broad in nature, overgeneralized, and distorted and can easily be tested and challenged through a series of behavioral experiments and by the use of straightforward

Negative beliefs about myself	Strength of belief (1–10)
1. I'm worthless.	10
2. I'm a terrible father.	10
3. I'm inflexible.	9
4. I don't have the ability to change.	9
5. I'm not creative.	8
Negative beliefs about others	**Strength of belief (1–10)**
1. Nobody cares about me.	10
2. Everybody criticizes me.	10
3. I don't have any real friends.	9
4. Everybody leaves me.	9
5. Nobody shows me any affection.	8

FIGURE 9.2. Hierarchy of beliefs about self and others from the suicidal belief system.

cognitive restructuring techniques (see later). Once put on paper, these characteristics become much more apparent to the patient.

In addition, keeping a list of the specific beliefs identified during therapy sessions provides a means to facilitate restructuring work. The beliefs can be placed in a hierarchy according to those that are most salient and problematic for the patient. The hierarchy can easily be established by simply asking the patient *how much he or she believes it to be true*, rating it on a scale of 1 to 10. Given that all beliefs are negative in quality and impact, the strength of the belief is likely the best characteristic on which to base the hierarchy. Once placed in the hierarchy, the patient can keep track of *how much* he or she *believes it* from session to session as treatment progresses, logging supporting or disconfirming evidence over time. This will be evidence uncovered during the course of sessions as well as evidence that is the direct result of subsequent behavioral experiments.

A Straightforward Strategy for Cognitive Change

Given its importance, we recommend using *a core set* of techniques and a standard approach regardless of the belief. This standard approach (i.e., the approach that the patient will learn to apply across episodes) can be supplemented, enhanced, and modified in the middle and later stages of treatment. The general approach recommended can easily be remembered by patient using the acronym ICARE—*I care*. The five steps can be written on a *coping card*, carried by the patient in a wallet or purse, and used frequently and with a fair degree of ease. It is best used in conjunction with an expanded STR, which provides the patient a permanent record of each incident and related intervention. The STR should be expanded to include the patient's restructured thought or belief, as well as the degree to which the patient believes it true after intervention (see Figure 9.3). This offers patients a means of keeping track of change over time, reorganizing their suicidal belief system belief hierarchy as needed. The following sequence of steps comprise the ICARE intervention method:

1. *Identify.* Identify the specific automatic thought and the underlying core belief. Write the thought/belief down on the expanded STR (see Figure 9.3). As reviewed previously, the identified thought or belief will ideally be on the patient's hierarchy. If not, it should be added to his or her running log and ranked accordingly. For example, as evidenced in Figure 9.3 the patient detailed the following: "I thought I was worthless and didn't deserve to live."

2. *Connect* the automatic thought to the distortion. Identify the distortion inherent to the belief (see Figure 9.4). Having the patient commit to memory

Triggering event(s)[A]	Suicidal thoughts[B]	Severity[C] (1–10)	Duration[D] (1–10)	Feelings[E]	Severity (1–10)	Duration (1–10)	Behavioral response[F]	Change[G] +/–
Had an argument with my wife. She left and I was at home alone.	I thought I was worthless, didn't deserve to live.	9	20 minutes.	Anger, frustration, sadness.	9	About 15 minutes.	I completed my STR, finished the ICARE response.	I'm not worthless, just upset.

My most common distortions:

Catastrophizing, emotional reasoning, magnification/minimization, personalization.

[A]Provide as much detail as possible. Indicate the full context, what day, time, who was present, what happened, and what did you do?
[B]Describe the specific thought(s) you had at the time. For example, "I thought of taking an overdose, that I didn't deserve to live, everybody would be better off if I was dead".
[C]Describe the intensity or severity of your thoughts on a scale of 1–10, with 1 being mild and 10 overwhelming.
[D]Note how long the thoughts lasted, a few seconds, minutes, hours, or days. Please try to be precise.
[E]Describe your feelings such as anger, sadness, guilt, anxiety. Remember, you can feel more than one thing at a time.
[F]Complete the ICARE steps.
[G]Rate the degree to which you believe the new belief (rating on a scale of 1–10).

FIGURE 9.3. Example of a completed expanded Suicidal Thought Record/self-monitoring sheet for cognitive restructuring.

the number of possible distortions listed in Figure 9.4 is probably unrealistic, particularly given that we (clinicians) cannot always recall distortions without a prompt. Just as with the hierarchy of beliefs, there are likely to be a few consistent distortions in which the patient engages across episodes of suicidality. A careful review of the patient's prior episodes will help the clinician identify those distortions that are most frequent. We recommend identifying three, but probably no more than four, to ensure that the intervention is feasible. The patient can amend the bottom of the STR to keep track of his or her most common distortions (see the bottom portion of the STR in Figure 8.3). In the example provided earlier, the patient identified the following distortions: *emotional reasoning, personalization, and magnification/minimization.*

3. *Assess* (evaluate) the thought/belief. A standard and fairly simple approach is recommended here. What is the evidence for/against the belief? Are there other possible reasons/explanations for the situation/circumstance? What is the worst thing that could happen? The best? The most likely? Will it matter in a year? In the example provided for Figure 9.3, the patient evaluated the belief in the following manner: "The *only* evidence for it is that my wife said some mean things because she was so upset and mad at me [limited evidence for the belief and another possible explanation]. Now that I think about it, I've done a lot of things in my life. I'm a good friend, a good father, and I'm trying as a husband [evidence against the belief]. The worst thing that could happen is that my wife could be gone for a few hours and come home still mad. She'd probably get over it by morning; she always has [most likely outcome]. Anyway, none of this will matter in a few days" [decatastrophizing].

4. *Restructure.* Restate the belief after having effectively evaluated it. What is a more reasonable alternative belief once the distortion has been removed and the belief decatastrophized? What are the advantages of giving up the dysfunctional suicidal belief identified? After careful evaluation, the patient in the example provided for Figure 8.3 restructured the belief in the following way: "I'm not worthless just upset that my wife said some mean things and hurt my feelings. I'll get over it, we'll make up as usual, and the world will go on. There's no reason to want to kill myself. I already feel better just writing this."

5. *Execute* (respond). Act as though the new belief were true. As is the case for many suicidal patients, there is often little logic or reasoning to negative core beliefs. They are frequently rooted in developmental trauma and a complex individual history, of which the emotional power is formidable. This is, in many ways, consistent with *emotional conditioning* (i.e., a suicidal, self-destructive, or self-defeating behavioral response secondary solely to a chronic negative emotion), something inherent to personality psychopathology. Acting on the restated belief provides an emotional experience to counter this process. Have the patient identify a set of steps/behaviors that are consistent with the restated belief. These will form the basis for a behavioral

Although some automatic thoughts are true, many are either untrue or have just a grain of truth. Typical mistakes in thinking include:

1. All-or-nothing thinking (also called black-and-white, polarized, or dichotomous thinking): You view a situation in only two categories instead of on a continuum.
   Example: "If I'm not a total success, I'm a failure."

2. Catastrophizing (also called fortune telling): You predict the future negatively without considering other, more likely outcomes.
   Example: "I'll be so upset, I won't be able to function at all."

3. Disqualifying or discounting the positive: You unreasonably tell yourself that positive experiences, deeds, or qualities do not count.
   Example: "I did that project well, but that doesn't mean I'm competent; I just got lucky."

4. Emotional reasoning: You think something must be true because you "feel" (actually believe) it so strongly, ignoring or discounting evidence to the contrary.
   Example: "I know I do a lot of things okay at work, but I still feel like I'm a failure."

5. Labeling: You put a fixed, global label on yourself or others without considering that the evidence might be more reasonably lead to a less disastrous conclusion.
   Example: "I'm a loser. He's no good."

6. Magnification/minimization: When you evaluate yourself, another person, or a situation, you unreasonably magnify the negative and/or minimize the positive.
   Example: "Getting a mediocre evaluation proves how inadequate I am. Getting high marks doesn't mean I'm smart."

7. Mental filter (also called selective abstraction): You pay undue attention to one negative detail
   instead of seeing the whole picture.
   Example: "Because I got one low rating on my evaluation (which also contained several high ratings) it means I'm doing a lousy job."

8. Mind reading: You believe you know what others are thinking, failing to consider other, more
   likely possibilities.
   Example: "He's thinking that I don't know the first thing about this project."

9. Overgeneralization: You make a sweeping negative conclusion that goes far beyond the current
   situation.
   Example: (Because I felt uncomfortable at the meeting) "I don't have what it takes to make friends."

(continued)

FIGURE 9.4. Common cognitive distortions handout. Adapted from Beck and Freeman (1990). Reprinted with permission.

10. Personalization: You believe others are behaving negatively because of you, without considering more plausible explanations for their behavior.
    Example: "The repairman was curt to me because I did something wrong."
11. "Should" and "must" statements (also called imperatives): You have a precise, fixed idea of how you or others should behave and you overestimate how bad it is that these expectations are not met.
    Example: "It's terrible that I made a mistake. I should always do my best."
12. Tunnel vision: You only see the negative aspects of a situation.
    Example: "My son's teacher can't do anything right. He's critical and insensitive and lousy at teaching."

FIGURE 9.4. *(cont.)*

experiment that can be used as further evidence to disconfirm long-standing negative core beliefs. After the behavioral experiment, the new belief can be rated once again (see column G in Figure 9.3). If problem solving is required, a specific approach is offered in Chapter 10. The patient described in Figure 8.3 decided to do the following: "When my wife gets home, I'm going to ask her to sit down and talk and try to identify what the problem really is. I'm also going to apologize for the things I said that hurt her feelings."

Naturally, implementing these steps will require the use of a broad range of intervention techniques common to cognitive therapy (questioning the evidence, reattribution, understanding idiosyncratic meaning, decatastrophizing, cost–benefit analysis, labeling distortions, scaling, thought stopping, guided discovery, Socratic questioning, self-instruction), as well as an active effort to help the patient develop a set of specific *life skills.* Consistent with the model emphasized in Chapter 10, we recommend an approach that is specific, simple, and accessible. Hence, the five-step model provided. Regardless of patient complexity or chronicity, we have found that two characteristics frequently predict success: *consistency and repetition.* The clinician likely will use a range of intervention techniques in the course of sessions targeting cognitive change, but at the heart of cognitive therapy is the use of skillful Socratic questioning and guided discovery. It is important not to do the patient's work for him or her but to help the patient link and explore what to date may have been viewed as disparate events. Following is an example of guided discovery with Mr. G, using simple questions such as "What happened next?" "What was going through your mind?" "How did you feel?" and "What did you end up doing?"

PATIENT [in midsession]: I don't know. I was just leaving the office and had the thought "I should kill myself."

THERAPIST: Did anything upsetting happen during the day? Anything stressful going on prior to that?

PATIENT: Well, nothing that I really paid much attention to. Earlier in the day, though, I had this patient that told me she wasn't getting anywhere and thought she should see another therapist.

THERAPIST: What went through your head when she said that?

PATIENT: I thought that I really didn't know what I was doing. I thought I probably should get out of the profession since I'm so incompetent. I can't see myself doing anything else; I've spent so long learning this stuff that I might as well die.

THERAPIST: Do you remember how you felt at the time?

PATIENT: Terrible. I got really depressed. It wasn't long after that when I got in my car and drove off, first I went to the bar and then out to the lake.

Dealing with Poor Motivation and Treatment Noncompliance

If the patient is not motivated to carry coping cards, complete STRs, or keep a running treatment log, a number of steps can be taken to encourage the patient to more actively participate in the treatment process. First, the patient's commitment-to-treatment statement needs to be reviewed and discussed (see Chapter 8). The patient's potential ambivalence about living and recovery needs to be explored. If the patient is not adequately motivated for treatment, it simply will not work. Second, the thoughts/beliefs regarding treatment noncompliance need to be specifically articulated and evaluated using the five-step model referenced earlier (e.g., *It's too much trouble to do the writing, I just don't have time, I'm too busy. Writing this stuff down is stupid!*). Specifically, the advantages/disadvantages of maintaining the noncompliance (and related beliefs) can be explored and examined in detail. A range of additional techniques can also be used as alternatives to writing, constrained only by the creativity of the clinician. We have found that encouraging patients to use audiotapes is highly effective and, often, provides a transition to writing. Use of audiotapes can be enhanced by routinely taping therapy sessions (both video and audio) and providing the tapes for the patient to review at home.

Evaluating the effectiveness of conditional rules and assumptions may take a little different approach. In many ways, the patient's conditional rules and assumptions form the foundation of what can be thought of as a *life phi-*

losophy. The lives of suicidal patients are constrained by a range of dysfunctional, punitive, self-destructive, and self-defeating *rules for living* that, during the height of a suicidal crisis, are simply unbearable.

Building a Philosophy for Living: Change and Acceptance as New Rules

To ensure lasting change, the patient will likely need to challenge his or her fundamental *philosophy of life.* Essentially, the patient's philosophy has not been *reasonable* or *livable,* incorporating a set of conditional rules and assumptions that are inflexible, rigid, simply ineffective, often grossly distorted, and frequently punitive. Even if triggered and a problem only *occasionally,* they are associated with feelings and behavior that clearly threaten the patient's emotional, and possibly physical, well-being. During the course of treatment, it is helpful to have the patient keep a list of new rules and assumptions as they emerge, providing a new *philosophy for living*: one that is flexible, reasonable, and compassionate. If the patient's new rules and assumptions are kept as a part of the ongoing treatment log (or simply jotted down on the STRs), they can be frequently reviewed, updated, or amended as needed.

Evaluating conditional rules and assumptions necessitates a somewhat different approach. Specifically, it is probably most effective to conduct repetitive *cost-benefit analyses* of rules and assumptions (and the compensatory strategy they define) as they emerge. Simply reviewing, in concrete terms, the advantages and disadvantages of a particular rule/assumption can do this. For example, in the case of Mr. G, perfectionism was employed in response to long-standing feelings of inadequacy and incompetence. Careful review, however, revealed for Mr. G that not only was perfectionism *not attainable and completely unrealistic* (disadvantage) but maintaining it as a standard *guaranteed that he would feel like a failure each and every day because he would never achieve his goal* (disadvantage). After careful review, Mr. G was unable to identify any advantages of maintaining his perfectionism. Initially, he proposed that "it helps me perform better," but after careful evaluation, this was discovered to be inaccurate. Mr. G actually realized that the goal of perfectionism probably inhibited his performance secondary to *feeling so pressured and stressed all the time.* It is important to remember that each review should be followed by a behavioral experiment in which the patient implements the new rule/assumption/standard. This provides an opportunity for direct comparison, quick evaluation of its effectiveness, and ready reinforcement for the patient. In the case of Mr. G, he noted that after a week of work with the new standard, that he felt *like a huge weight had*

been lifted from his shoulders. He reported that work was much more re-
warding and that he was *more efficient.*

As noted previously, central to the idea of developing a new *philosophy
for living* is establishing a more functional and healthier set of conditional
rules and assumptions for daily living. Inherent to any *set of rules* for living
is the issue of acceptance. Hayes (1987) has fashioned *acceptance and commitment therapy*, an approach that offers *psychological acceptance* as a central coping strategy. This therapeutic approach encourages patients to *accept*
the inevitability of occasional painful, negative emotional experiences (e.g.,
developmentally based painful emotions, distressing memories, and upsetting physical sensations). They are encouraged to recognize that occasional
painful experiences alone do not prevent an enjoyable and productive life,
nor does the occasional recurrence of a painful emotion signal treatment
failure.

Acceptance, in some form or fashion, is important to integrate into the
patient's *new* philosophy for living. Acceptance can be defined in a simple
fashion for the patient. It is the acknowledgment and recognition, both emotionally and through our behavior (conduct), of things over which we can exert
no control (e.g., the behavior of others or random events). Simply put, when
someone accepts something, they stop acting as if they can change it. As viv-
idly illustrated in Figure 9.5, this issue will likely emerge as the patient starts
to articulate new rules and assumptions for daily living. Ideally, they will be
ones that are more forgiving, reasonable, and compassionate. Inherent to
many of them will be *acceptance.* This is also a critical component of the
skills training discussed in Chapter 10, particularly distress tolerance and
problem solving. In many respects, the skills training detailed in Chapter 10
will help the patient develop and refine his or her ability to *accept* certain
things about the nature of living.

After careful evaluation, much time and effort, I've decided to implement the
following rules for my life:

1. Accept the fact that I'm not perfect and never will be.
2. Do the best job I can and feel good about it.
3. Recognize the things I do well each and every day.
4. Identify and work on accepting the things I cannot change, in myself,
    others, and the world around me.
5. Accept the fact that bad things are going to happen to me and I need to
    learn to deal better with them when they do.

FIGURE 9.5. An example of a patient's "Philosophy for Living" statement.

Prevailing, Facilitating, and Compensatory Modes in Chronic Suicidality: Developing Adaptive Modes and Acknowledging Personal Qualities and Characteristics

It is important to keep in mind that for those who are chronically suicidal, the majority of the work will target prevailing and facilitating compensatory modes. Facilitating modes are those that incorporate cognitions, affect, and behavior that *heighten the risk* for activation of the suicidal mode. These are the compensatory modes that are present the majority of the time (prevailing in nature), that is, when the patient is not actively suicidal. The cognitive restructuring discussed in this chapter facilitates change, but in order to effect lasting change, the chronic patient needs to develop more *adaptive modes*. More adaptive modes are essentially represented by a restructured suicidal belief system, with identifiable and observable change in beliefs about self, others, and the future. Depending on the type of prominent Axis II traits present, the content of the suicidal belief system will vary from individual to individual. Beck, Freeman, and Associates (1990) have provided a list of *typical* beliefs about self and others for each specific personality disorder.

We have found that the most effective way to target and effect change in self-image and, accordingly, facilitate the development of more adaptive modes is to have the patient keep a list of his or her active beliefs about self and others as a part of the treatment log. Adaptive modes are those that *facilitate recovery and heighten the probability of successful adaptation*. We encourage patients to journal for anywhere from 5 to 30 minutes a day. As a part of this activity, the patient is encouraged to *keep a tab* of these beliefs on a daily basis, listing interactions, situations, and circumstances that confirm or disconfirm (i.e., evidence for and against) the beliefs. This idea is similar to that of the *core belief worksheet* proposed by Beck (1995). Naturally, changing these beliefs will take time, often months to years. Strategically planned behavioral experiments can be used to reinforce the emergence of particular traits (see Chapter 10).

As was noted in the treatment-planning matrix offered in Chapter 3, self-image change requires considerably more time. Nonetheless, much of the work necessary for lasting self-image change occurs in the context of skill building. As discussed in Chapter 10, most skills require an interpersonal context and provide an opportunity to address beliefs about self and others quite effectively. This points to the need to conceptualize each treatment component as interdependent and overlapping. Although the clinician may be focusing on *one specific goal at a time*, he or she is more than likely addressing issues that cut across all three components, just to varying degrees.

The Therapeutic Belief System: Therapy-Specific Beliefs

The therapeutic belief system is a way for the therapist to understand, organize, discuss, and ultimately address aspects of the therapeutic relationship in CBT, consistent with the fundamental principles of cognitive therapy summarized by Clark (1995). In other words, the therapeutic belief system is a way for the clinician to organize and discuss therapy-specific beliefs that fall into three domains: (1) beliefs about the therapist, (2) beliefs about the treatment process, and (3) beliefs about the patient's role in treatment. Simply put, it allows the therapist to (1) diagram the patient's (and therapist's) active beliefs, assumptions, and automatic thoughts about the therapeutic process; (2) understand the patient's (and therapist's) explicit and implicit emotional and behavioral responses; and (3) identify specific targets to facilitate a productive relationship and better treatment outcome. It is also consistent with the cognitive case conceptualization framework recently offered by Beck (1995) and mentioned in Chapter 1.

If the therapeutic belief system can be accurately defined then, ideally, the therapeutic relationship itself can be maximized as a vehicle of change and potential treatment resistance (and provocations) can be undermined and responded to openly and effectively. This is particularly true in terms of addressing issues related to core cognitive structures and underlying schemas, those most resistant to change (see Chapter 2). Few relationships offer the potency and intensity, regardless of duration, as does a therapeutic encounter in the treatment of suicidality. In addition, the potential for productive and healthy implicit learning via the process of covariation (e.g., Reber, 1992) in a therapeutic relationship is significant. Accordingly, the potential for productive, effective, and lasting change at multiple levels is profound if an accurate conceptualization and organization of the clinical material about the therapeutic relationship can be accomplished.

The therapeutic belief system incorporates beliefs that revolve around three identifiable components of the therapeutic process including (1) the therapist, (2) the patient, and (3) the nature of treatment itself. In other words, a therapeutic belief system diagram can be outlined for each component part. Naturally, conceptualizations of the therapeutic belief system may differ between patient and therapist but ideally would be complementary. If not, this would clearly be a clinical issue to address in treatment, much as would be the case with conflicting goals or markers of treatment progress between patient and therapist. As detailed in Figure 9.6, different beliefs, assumptions, and automatic thoughts regarding the therapist (as seen by the patient) will result in different emotional and behavioral responses, each representing an identifiable treatment target consistent with the conceptualization of the suicidal mode offered in Chapter 2. The additional components of Figure 9.6 provide examples for the patient/self beliefs and the patient's view of the treatment

A. TREATMENT COMPONENT: THERAPIST (AS SEEN BY PATIENT)

1. Active core belief(s) about therapist:

Themes:
   Victimizer: "He/she is going to hurt me, reject me, or abandon me."
   Collaborator: "He/she is going to work with me, help me."
   Savior: "He/she is going to protect me, save me."

2. Active assumption(s) about therapist:

Themes:
   Victimizer: "If I open up and let him/her close, I'm going to get hurt, rejected, or abandoned."
   Collaborator: "If I work with him/her, I'll do better."
   Savior: "If I just come to treatment, he/she will do what's necessary to protect me, save me."

3. Active compensatory strategy(ies):

Themes:
   Victimizer: active resistance.
   Collaborator: active participation.
   Savior: passive resistance.

4. Example of identifiable automatic thoughts:

Themes:
   Victimizer: "Nobody cares about me, everyone's out for themselves."
   Collaborator: "Maybe somebody can help me."
   Savior: "I need someone to take care of me."

5. Emotional response(s):

Themes:
   Victimizer: anger, hostility, fear, rage, hypervigilance, hate.
   Collaborator: hopefulness, anxiety.
   Savior: apprehension, depression, anxiety.

6. Behavioral response(s):

Themes:
   Victimizer: hostile, aggressive/provocative acting out (e.g., argumentative, self-destructive behavior).
   Collaborator: active participation.
   Savior: passivity, reassurance seeking, prominent dependency.

B. TREATMENT COMPONENT: PATIENT/SELF

1. Active core belief(s) about self:

Themes:
   Victim: "I'm vulnerable, helpless."
   Collaborator: "I can work with someone to improve, do better."
   Caretaker: " I don't deserve help, others do."

(continued)

FIGURE 9.6. Example of the therapeutic belief system. Adapted from Rudd & Joiner (1997). Used by permission of Springer Publishing Company, Inc., New York 10012.

2. Active assumption(s) about self:

Themes:
> **Victim:** "If I don't let myself be vulnerable, I'll be OK."
> **Collaborator:** "If I work with someone I can improve, do better."
> **Caretaker:** "If I take care of others, I'll feel better."

3. Active compensatory strategy(ies):

Themes:
> **Victim:** passive or active resistance (e.g., withdrawal, passivity vs. provocative acting out).
> **Collaborator:** active participation.
> **Caretaker:** caretaking, external focus, focus on others (e.g., therapist).

4. Example of identifiable automatic thoughts:

Themes:
> **Victim:** "I'll get hurt if I open up."
> **Collaborator:** "I can do better if we work together."
> **Caretaker:** " Others deserve help more than me."

5. Emotional response(s):

Themes:
> **Victim:** hopelessness, helplessness, depression, anxiety, hypervigilance.
> **Collaborator:** hopefulness, anxiety.
> **Caretaker:** apprehension, depression, anxiety

6. Behavioral response(s):

Themes:
> **Victim:** passive resistance (e.g., withdrawal and limited participation) vs. active resistance (e.g., acting-out behaviors).
> **Collaborator:** active participation.
> **Caretaker:** caretaking, comforting.

C. TREATMENT COMPONENT: TREATMENT PROCESS (AS SEEN BY PATIENT)

1. Active core belief (s) about treatment:

Themes:
> **Hopeless:** "Treatment is hopeless."
> **Maintenance:** "Treatment will maintain status quo, get by, but I won't do better."
> **Productive:** " Treatment can help me improve, solve problems, do better."

2. Active assumption(s) about treatment:

Themes:
> **Hopeless:** "If I try, it won't make any difference."
> **Maintenance:** "If I try, things will just stay the same."
> **Productive:** " If I try, I can improve, solve my problems, do better."

(continued)

FIGURE 9.6. *(cont.)*

3. Active compensatory strategy(ies):

Themes:
    Hopeless: early withdrawal, inactivity (e.g., not completing homework, other therapeutic activities).
    Maintenance: limited, guarded effort.
    Productive: active participation.

4. Example of identifiable automatic thoughts:

Themes:
    Hopeless: "This is pointless, nothing will help."
    Maintenance: "Thing will just stay the same."
    Productive: " There are some options, solutions."

5. Emotional response(s):

Themes:
    Hopeless: despair, hopelessness, helpless, depression, anxiety.
    Maintenance: pessimism, cynicism, depression, anxiety.
    Productive: hopefulness, anxiety.

6. Behavioral response(s):

    Themes:
    Hopeless: quitting treatment, not completing homework.
    Maintenance: limited activity.
    Productive: active participation.

D. TREATMENT COMPONENT: PATIENT (AS SEEN BY THERAPIST)

1. Active core belief(s) about patient:

Themes:
    Hostile Aggressor: "He or she is only trouble, a threat to me professionally."
    Collaborator: "He or she is capable and going to work with me to help him- or herself."
    Helpless Victim: "He or she is incapable of taking care of him- or herself or actively working toward a solution to the problem."

2. Active assumption(s) about patient:

Themes:
    Hostile Aggressor: "If I treat him or her, it could ruin my practice."
    Collaborator: "If I work with this patient, he or she will probably improve."
    Helpless Victim: "If I don't do more for this patient, he or she will get worse."

3. Active compensatory strategy(ies):

Themes:
    Hostile Aggressor: rejection, abandonment (e.g., through referral).
    Collaborator: active treatment.
    Helpless Victim: overprotective, caretaking, meddling intervention.

(continued)

FIGURE 9.6. *(cont.)*

---

4. Example of identifiable automatic thoughts:

Themes:

    Hostile Aggressor: "He/she could ruin my practice."

    Collaborator: "He/she is working hard, trying."

    Helpless Victim: "He/she can't take on too much right now."

---

5. Emotional response(s):

Themes:

    Hostile Aggressor: anger, hate, rage, fear, apprehension, anxiety, hopelessness.

    Collaborator: hopefulness, anxiety.

    Helpless Victim: apprehension, anxiety, sadness, depression.

---

6. Behavioral response(s):

Themes:

    Hostile Aggressor: termination of treatment, referral, provocative behavior (e.g., being late for appointments, cancellations, confrontational and blaming patient).

    Collaborator: active treatment.

    Helpless Victim: overly cautious monitoring, caretaking, more frequent visits, lower threshold for hospitalization, frequent intervention.

E. TREATMENT COMPONENT: THERAPIST/SELF

---

1. Active core belief(s) about self:

Themes:

    Victim: "I'm vulnerable, inadequate, incompetent."

    Collaborator: "If we work together, I can help this patient, I'm competent, capable."

    Savior: " Only I can help this patient."

---

2. Active assumption(s) about self:

Themes:

    Victim: "If I protect myself, I'll be OK, others won't see my incompetence, inadequacy."

    Collaborator: "If I do what I know, I can facilitate a good treatment collaboration and outcome."

    Savior: "If I don't do everything, for this patient treatment will fail."

---

3. Active compensatory strategy(ies):

Themes:

    Victim: active resistance, defensive posturing (e.g., argumentative, confrontational, and blaming patient), outright rejection, abandonment through refusal to treat, referral.

    Collaborator: active participation.

    Savior: caretaking, overly active, meddling intervention, close and unnecessary monitoring.

(continued)

FIGURE 9.6. *(cont.)*

---

4. Example of identifiable automatic thoughts:

Themes:
>   **Victim:** "I'll get hurt if I work with this patient."
>   **Collaborator:** "I can work effectively with this patient."
>   **Savior:** " Without me he/she won't make it."

---

5. Emotional response(s):

Themes:
>   **Victim:** hopelessness, helplessness, depression, anxiety, hypervigilance, anger, hate, rage, fear.
>   **Collaborator:** hopefulness, anxiety.
>   **Savior:** apprehension, depression, anxiety.

---

6. Behavioral response(s):

Themes:
>   **Victim:** termination of treatment, referral, provocative behavior (e.g., being late for appointments, cancellations, confrontational, and blaming patient).
>   **Collaborator:** active participation.
>   **Savior:** overly cautious monitoring, caretaking, more frequent visits, lower threshold for hospitalization, meddling and unnecessary interventions.

F. TREATMENT COMPONENT: TREATMENT PROCESS (AS SEEN BY THERAPIST)

---

1. Active core belief(s) about treatment:

Themes:
>   **Hopeless:** "Treatment is hopeless."
>   **Maintenance:** "Treatment will help me keep status quo, get by, but he or she won't do better."
>   **Productive:** " Treatment can help him/her improve, solve their problems, do better."

---

2. Active assumption(s) about treatment:

Themes:
>   **Hopeless:** "If I try, treatment won't make any difference."
>   **Maintenance:** "If I try, things will just stay the same."
>   **Productive:** " If I try, treatment can make a difference."

---

3. Active compensatory strategy(ies):

Themes:
>   **Hopeless:** treatment termination, referral to another provider.
>   **Maintenance:** limited, guarded effort (e.g., poor conceptualization and no clear goals).
>   **Productive:** active participation.

(continued)

FIGURE 9.6. *(cont.)*

---

4. Example of identifiable automatic thoughts:

Themes:
  Hopeless: "This is pointless, nothing will help."
  Maintenance: "Thing will just stay the same."
  Productive: " There are some options, solutions."

---

5. Emotional response(s):

Themes:
  Hopeless: despair, hopelessness, depression, anxiety.
  Maintenance: pessimism, cynicism, depression, anxiety.
  Productive: hopefulness, anxiety.

---

6. Behavioral response(s):

Themes:
  Hopeless: treatment termination, referral to another provider.
  Maintenance: limited activity, effort (e.g., poor conceptualization and no clear
    goals).
  Productive: active participation.

FIGURE 9.6. *(cont.)*

process in general. The possible clinical examples are innumerable and vary from patient to patient and across a broad range of variables (e.g., Axis I and II diagnoses, comorbidity, presenting problems, developmental history, educational and occupational history, previous treatment experiences). The examples provided detail some commonly encountered themes with suicidal patients, the implications of which are discussed in more detail in the following sections.

Outlining the Therapeutic Belief System

Completing the therapeutic belief system is simple and straightforward. To do so, the therapist needs the following information: a list of the patient's core beliefs about treatment (including the therapist, the treatment process, and his or her role), active assumptions about treatment, active compensatory strategies, identifiable automatic thoughts, routine emotional responses, and frequent behavioral responses. Most of this information is readily available from the suicidal mode that has already been completed. Sometimes, though, it will be necessary to question the patient about therapy-specific beliefs. The therapeutic belief system simply provides the clinician a way to organize aspects of the suicidal mode and facilitating modes that weigh heavily on the therapeutic relationship and treatment process.

Three simple steps can be followed in completing the therapeutic belief system (a separate diagram is done for each category of core beliefs: therapist, self, and treatment process):

1. Access the previously articulated suicidal mode.
2. If specific treatment-related beliefs are not available, discuss with the patient his or her perception of the treatment process, the role of the therapist in treatment, and the patient's role in treatment.
3. Organize each component part in hierarchical fashion moving from core beliefs, active assumptions, compensatory strategies, automatic thoughts, and emotional response, to behavioral responses.

Therapeutic belief system diagrams can be used in any number of ways. Perhaps, most important, though, the diagrams can be used to facilitate the discussion of the therapeutic relationship. The therapeutic belief system diagram provides a concrete illustration of how therapy-related beliefs affect the patient's behavior and, ultimately, treatment outcome. It is recommended that when they are used, they be made part of the permanent clinical record.

Figure 9.6 provides an example of common themes in the therapeutic belief system for suicidal patients. As illustrated, active beliefs about the therapist are described as shifting along a continuum from a potential victimizer to collaborator/partner to savior. Each shift brings with it unique core beliefs, assumptions, automatic thoughts, and associated emotional and behavioral responses. Naturally, the ideal is for the patient to view the therapist as collaborator, consistent with the fundamental principles of cognitive therapy and a more effective treatment process. However, if there is a shift in either direction, the therapeutic belief system offers explanatory clinical material and rich treatment targets, all of which can be actively pursued with the patient. Similarly, the patient's view of self is described as shifting along a continuum from victim to collaborator to caretaker. Again, each theme carries with it a belief system with unique emotional and behavioral consequences. Finally, the conceptualization of the treatment process itself is described as varying along a continuum from hopeless to maintenance to productive change. Figure 9.6 provides a summary of the patient's response to each identifiable component of the treatment process, detailing what has been referred to in the psychodynamic literature as transference reactions. However, the framework provided is inherently more consistent with a cognitive conceptualization and, accordingly, offers a wealth of clinical material that can be directly targeted in treatment with traditional cognitive therapy techniques (particularly cognitive restructuring, discussed in Chapter 9).

The therapeutic belief system can also be completed for the clinician, detailing the therapist's response(s) to each treatment component. As illustrated in Figure 9.6, the clinician's response(s) to the suicidal patient may vary along a continuum from hostile aggressor to receptive collaborator to helpless victim. Each case will result in varying assumptions, automatic thoughts, and related emotional and behavioral responses, all ripe for clinical intervention. Similarly, the identifiable themes for the therapist's view of self are victim, collaborator, and savior. Finally, the themes for the therapist's view of the treatment process vary from hopeless to maintenance to productive change.

It is not uncommon in clinical practice to have patients who will readily voice hope and optimism regarding treatment and experience positive, identifiable, and even quantifiable gains yet report profound emotional discomfort, dysphoria, and difficulty associated with the therapeutic process. It is possible that a range of tacit beliefs and associated emotions are triggered by the intimacy and intensity of the therapeutic process. It is assumed that the defining feature of tacit beliefs is that they are outside the range of conscious awareness. For example, if it were a suicidal patient with an early history of abuse, the therapeutic encounter itself (simply due to the level of intimacy inherent in the process) might trigger tacit beliefs of mistrust and vulnerability as well as associated anxiety, anger, apprehension, shame, and dysphoria which could lead to the patient's withdrawal from treatment (i.e., compensatory strategy). Along these lines, Rudd et al. (1995) found that premature withdrawal from treatment appeared to be secondary to such interpersonal hypersensitivity and that withdrawal occurred despite the fact that patients' continued to be highly symptomatic and in distress. Although patients may not be able to consciously articulate such beliefs, or recognize the emergence of subtle compensatory withdrawal strategies, they may voice strong emotional reactions which at a surface level are difficult for the therapist to understand. To dismiss the patient's emotional response as transference consistent with, for example, a borderline personality framework would be to miss a critical opportunity for clinical intervention, belief activation, and associated cognitive restructuring.

A clear cognitive conceptualization of potential *tacit beliefs* and related responses on the part of both the therapist and patient would enable the therapist to respond in a more clinically effective manner. In the previous example, the patient's clinical presentation could be compounded by the emergence of a therapist's tacit beliefs of failure and inadequacy. For example, the clinician might respond to the patient's anger, dysphoria, and resultant withdrawal behaviors by quickly discussing the need for referral to another provider. Such a response would only compound underlying themes of mistrust and vulnerability with abandonment. On the other hand, a clear conceptualization would help the clinician understand that the patient's emotional and behavioral responses are likely an indication of treatment *progress*, given that critical core beliefs and underlying schemas have been triggered and are amenable to modification or change even if in a limited fashion. Accordingly, the therapist might chose to be methodical, patient, persistent, not emotionally reactive, and repetitive. In other words, the therapist would more effectively manage what would have previously been termed "a countertransference reaction." Rather than pathologizing the patient's reaction, the cognitive therapist would likely view such resistance as a natural, a healthy, and an effective response given the patient's past traumatic history and experience (Mahoney, 1988b). Although eventual therapeutic change might well be a lengthy process, the focus in cognitive therapy would be on making the implicit explicit, taking advantage of a critical opportunity for cognitive restructuring regardless of how subtle.

It is recommended that the therapeutic belief system be detailed for each suicidal patient, particularly for those who are more provocative and resistant to treatment. The therapeutic belief system should complement the conceptual model offered in Chapter 2. In many respects, detailing the therapeutic belief system allows the therapist to more clearly understand active, potential, or even tacit treatment resistance by the patient and counterproductive interactions on the part of the therapist and provides a conceptual framework to answer many of the questions posed by Newman (1994) in his discussion of treatment resistance:

1. What is the function of the client's resistance behaviors?
2. How does the client's current resistance fit into his or her developmental/historical pattern of resistance?
3. What might be some of the client's idiosyncratic beliefs that are feeding into his or her resistance?
4. What might the client fear will happen if he or she complies?
5. How might the client be characteristically be misunderstanding or misinterpreting the therapists suggestions, methods, or intentions?
6. What skills does the client lack that might make it practically difficult or impossible at this point for him or her to actively collaborate with treatment?
7. What factors in the client's natural environment may be punishing the client's attempts to change?
8. Does the conceptualization of the case need to be revised or amended?

At a minimum, the therapeutic belief system offers specific treatment targets across multiple domains and, ideally, a more conceptually and theoretically consistent means of addressing concerns about what has been referred to as transference–countertransference reactions in cognitive therapy. Specifically, the therapeutic belief system does the following:

1. Ensures that the patient is an active participant in the definition of reality utilized during treatment.

2. Makes relevant cognition(s) knowable and accessible.
3. Emphasizes cognition as central to the therapeutic change process.
4. Creates opportunity for making the implicit explicit, recognizing the role of tacit beliefs and creating opportunity for associated cognitive restructuring.
5. Ensures a present time frame regardless of issues being addressed (i.e., even tacit beliefs and underlying schemas are addressed in terms of the current dysfunction created).

The Therapeutic Belief System of the Therapist Treating Suicidality: Monitoring Thoughts, Feelings, and Behaviors in Treatment

Figure 9.6 offers an example of the therapeutic belief system applied to a suicidal patient is offered in as a means of understanding the importance of the therapeutic relationship in the treatment of this population as well identifying particular problem areas. Consistent with Maltsberger and Buie's (1974, 1989) discussion of *countertransference hate,* the therapeutic belief system for the clinician that will inevitably result in the most significant clinical management problems with suicidal patients is one in which the therapist views the patient as a hostile aggressor, views him- or herself as a victim (or potential victim), and the treatment process in general as hopeless. The active or tacit beliefs (i.e., therapist's view of self) will most likely revolve around themes of vulnerability, inadequacy, and incompetence with the therapist's likely affective/emotional response being characterized by anger, hate, rage, fear, apprehension, anxiety, and hopelessness. If unrecognized and not clinically managed (i.e., tacit in nature), the end result may be the very act most feared by many suicidal patients, rejection or abandonment in some form or fashion with a concomitant reinforcement of the patient's view of self as inadequate, defective, or unlovable. Typical behaviors that may alert the clinician to potential rejection or abandonment compensatory strategies on his or her part include a quick decision to terminate treatment without adequate exploration of other treatment options/alternatives for the patient, quick referral to another provider (e.g., at the first sign of trouble or following a suicide attempt by the patient), or a host of potentially provocative behaviors (i.e., treatment disruptions) such as being late for appointments, recurrent cancellations or rescheduling on the part of the therapist, and a confrontational or blaming approach in the treatment process.

As Maltsberger and Buie (1974, 1989) have eloquently described, the provocative behavior of the suicidal and chronically suicidal patient can be unrelenting. The natural or most frequent response, particularly for the less experienced therapist, will be to see the patient as a hostile aggressor, him- or herself as a victim, and treatment as potentially hopeless. Although more subtle in nature, another identifiable theme can be potentially counterproductive in the treatment of suicidal patients. Specifically, the therapist viewing the patient as a helpless victim, him- or herself as savior, and the treatment process as the only solution to the patient's problems can ultimately lead to overprotective and caretaking behavior, lower threshold for hospitalization, and meddling and unnecessary interventions on the part of the therapist. The end result for the patient may simply be a facilitation of prominent dependency, without adequate development of adaptive coping skills. An additional consequence can be the emergence of significant boundary problems, all too common with this population, such as frequent and demanding telephone calls, more frequent appointments, longer duration of treatment appointments, and, paradoxically, more severe acting-out behavior (e.g., attempts and self-mutilatory behavior) when the clinician attempts to reestablish appropriate therapeutic boundaries (e.g., Linehan, 1993).

In the treatment of suicidal patients, the therapeutic belief system offers clinicians a means to organize such potentially destructive core beliefs (i.e., both active and tacit), related automatic thoughts, compensatory strategies, and emotional and behavioral correlates in a coherent fashion. Such organization will ideally facilitate more effective clinical management, through either individual assessment or consultation. At a minimum, it provides a means for clinicians to clearly articulate therapeutic relationship variables, critical to the treatment of suicidal patients, in a manner consistent with the fundamental principles of cognitive therapy.

In summary, it is recommended that clinicians use the therapeutic belief system in the following manner:

1. Complete a therapeutic belief system for themselves with each suicidal patient with whom they work. It will vary as patients vary.
2. Check that the therapeutic belief system complements their conceptual model for the patient. There should be consistency between the two.
3. Identify any potential problematic beliefs (e.g., seeing themselves as the patient's *savior*), emotional responses, and behaviors.
4. Target identified problem areas using traditional CBT techniques (see Chapters 6–10).
5. Integrate identified problems into the discussion of the therapeutic relationship as needed. That is, clearly articulate the boundaries and realities of treatment (e.g., that the clinician *cannot protect or save the patient, or can the clinician solve the patient's problems*).
6. Seek consultation or supervision as needed. The importance and value of supervision and consultation is clear. It is a resource that, all too often, is not accessed.

Evaluating the Relationship: Patience, Determination, and Consistency

As mentioned earlier, it is important to actively monitor the therapeutic relationship. The therapeutic belief system provides a way to do this. In addition, the clinician can use the *Therapeutic Beliefs Scale* (TBS) periodically to evaluate the nature and quality of the therapy process (see Figure 9.7). The TBS has three factors: (1) beliefs about the therapeutic alliance (i.e., agreement about conceptualization and interventions), (2) beliefs about therapeutic skillfulness, and (3) beliefs about the interpersonal skills of the therapist (i.e., warmth, sincerity, empathy, and genuineness). Figure 9.7 lists the items that comprise each factor. The scale is relatively short and easy to use and interpret and can be used repeatedly during the course of treatment. The clinician simply adds the items for a total score. Also he or she can look at the three factors separately to address different aspects of the therapeutic relationship and alliance, as well as to conceptualize the therapeutic belief system (for both clinician and patient). We recommend use of the scale in strategic fashion, perhaps on a monthly basis. Clearly it should be used early in the treatment process, even after the first session if acute dysphoria and upset have adequately resolved.

Instructions: Please check how strongly you believe each of the following statements to be true about your most recent therapy session.	0—Not at all true	1—Somewhat true	2—Moderately true	3—Completely true
1. My therapist has defined my problems correctly.				
2. My therapist is doing the right things to help me with my problems.				
3. My therapist and I are working well together.				
4. My therapist understands what I am talking about.				
5. My therapist is helping me.				
6. I understand what my therapist says about my problems.				
7. My therapist has confidence in what he or she is doing.				
8. My therapist does the right things at the right times.				
9. My therapist cares about me and my life.				
10. My therapist is interested in helping me with difficult problems.				
11. I can tell my therapist anything and everything.				
12. My therapist is receptive to what I have to say.				
Total score (add columns 1–12)				Total score

Therapeutic Alliance Factor: Items 1, 3, 4, 6

Therapeutic Skillfulness Factor: Items 2, 5, 7, 8

Interpersonal Relatedness Factor: Items 9, 10, 11, 12

FIGURE 9.7. The Therapeutic Belief Scale. From *Treating Suicidal Behavior: An Effective, Time-Limited Approach* by M. David Rudd, Thomas Joiner, and M. Hasan Rajab. Copyright 2001 by The Guilford Press. Permission to reproduce this figure is granted to purchasers of this book for personal use only (see copyright page for details).

10

Skill Building: Developing Adaptive Modes and Ensuring Lasting Change

Conceptualizing Skill Deficits in Cognitive-Behavioral Therapy for Suicidality

This chapter discusses the six basic skill areas covered in the treatment-planning matrix described in Chapter 3. These six areas are by no means all inclusive. They simply represent those areas we have found most frequently deficient, and critically important, among those presenting with suicidality, both acute and chronic. The clinician can use any, or all, of the skill areas covered depending on the particular clinical presentation. The six basic skills discussed here can be viewed as individual *components* and implemented accordingly. This is frequently a necessity in a time-limited treatment environment. Naturally, however, there is some overlap in terms of content across the six areas, forming a basic *skill package* with each component part complementing the whole. From this perspective, the component parts are interdependent and deleting one may influence the effectiveness of another. Actually, this is an area that warrants considerable research attention. What component parts of the whole treatment package are actually effective, that is, what is *essential* to effective treatment? Because we have not yet answered some of the most fundamental questions about treatment efficacy with this population, however, this question is a bit premature.

Self-monitoring, distress tolerance, and emotion regulation are believed to be critical skills for all suicidal patients and represent *core interventions* that will be standard, regardless of the specific clinical presentation. This is primarily a function of the theoretical model that serves as the foundation of the CBT approach offered. All are essential for effective crisis intervention (see Chapter 6), accurately conceptualizing the patient's suicidal mode (see Chapter 2) and articulating the suicidal cycle for a specific episode (see Chapters 7 and 8). In other words, each skill is inherent to the very process of crisis intervention and case conceptualization within the CBT framework offered.

Occasionally, extreme time limitations allow only one or two additional components to be covered. In these cases, the efficacy of the intervention, particularly with respect to lasting gains, is naturally suspect. Under the most extreme time limitations, the clinician may only be able to address effective problem solving. For others, all six components will be possible and necessary for effective (and lasting) treatment. This is perhaps one of the primary advantages of the CBT theoretical framework provided: the ability to identify *component parts* of treatment and, accordingly, recognize implications for treatment delivery, outcome, and relapse. Included among the skill areas covered are the following (some of which have been discussed in previous chapters):

- Problem solving
- Emotion regulation
- Self-monitoring
- Distress tolerance
- Interpersonal skills (i.e., assertiveness)
- Anger management

Consistent with the discussion in Chapter 3, one of the primary goals of skill building is to identify the patient's skill deficits and target them accordingly. This is also consistent with the broader goal of enhancing the patient's overall adaptive coping and resiliency by modifying the structural content of the suicidal belief system. Nonetheless, it is important to keep in mind that each and every patient's needs will differ; some will require exposure to each and every content area in addition to the *core interventions*, some only one or two (primarily the result of severe external time constraints or limitations). Some will require *repeated* coverage of each and every content area over long time frames. In reality, though, many, if not all, of the content areas are likely to be addressed in psychotherapy, regardless of the specific skill deficiencies identified or the psychotherapeutic model employed. The vast majority of psychotherapy conducted today targets the content areas summarized previously in some form or fashion. We are simply advocating that this material be covered in a specific and concrete manner, that changes in skill level (+ or –) be monitored in a routine and predictable way, and subsequent treatment efforts vary accordingly (i.e., less vs. more [or repeated] time and attention).

Targeting Skill Deficits

Ensuring Understanding and Generating Motivation for Change

To facilitate effective skill building, the clinician needs to ensure that the patient understands its importance, agrees with the conceptual model offered, and is adequately motivated for change. Although discussing the suicidal mode and the suicidal cycle facilitates this process, the clinician needs to take a few additional steps to enhance the patient's understanding of the role of identified skill deficits. This is can be accomplished by doing the following:

1. Identify specific skill deficits for the patient in conjunction with reviewing the suicidal cycle. The clinician will want to make sure that the concept of skill deficits makes reasonable sense to the patient. In other words, the patient needs to see it as important enough to devote time and energy to change. The clinician should be sure to keep a running log of skill deficiencies (i.e., as a part of self-monitoring using the STR, treatment log, or daily journal). For example:

> "As we review your cycle, it looks like there are several problem areas we need to specifically target in treatment. For example, when you got angry at your boyfriend, you had trouble waiting before you did something, and then when you did, it was not only something that usually makes things worse (i.e., drinking), it was something that was self-destructive and ended up only hurting you. Actually, it hurt you in many different ways. You got sick [physical consequence], ended up in another fight [interpersonal consequence], and felt very guilty and ashamed the next day [emotional, self-image consequence]. This suggests that we need to emphasize work in several areas including distress tolerance (i.e., impulsivity), anger management, and problem solving."

If necessary, define each content area for the patient and provide specific examples to ensure adequate comprehension. Actually, asking the patient for an example is one of the most effective ways of ensuring adequate understanding. For example:

> "It sounds like you have a good grasp of what I'm suggesting are some of the problems. Can you think of another time that you've demonstrated poor distress tolerance? Tell me about it."

2. Place the deficit in context, both developmentally and with respect to current functioning (i.e., help the patient recognize and understand the implications of the deficit both in terms of previous problems and his or her current suicidal presentation). Placing the deficit *in context* makes it much more difficult for the patient to dismiss the suicidal episode as a *one time crisis, something that will never happen again*. In essence, it forces that patient to acknowledge a history of problems and difficulty even if not previously suicidal, while recognizing a variable critical for effective recovery (i.e., this step can *paradoxically* facilitate hopefulness). For example:

> "From what you've told me about your background and personal history, it sounds like these are things that you've struggled with for some time. I believe you mentioned that from an early age you've had trouble with anger, both in not feeling like you could tolerate it well and believing that you had to act 'immediately' or you would 'explode.' I believe you also mentioned that both your mother and father had problems controlling their anger and were frequently physically violent and verbally abusive during your childhood and adolescence. How many years would you say that you've struggled with these problems? Prior to coming in for treatment, do you believe things have gotten worse over the years, better, or stayed about the same?"

3. Identify, explore, and emphasize (if appropriate) the potentially recurrent nature of the problem or deficit over time. It is important to help the patient link recurrent episodes around a common theme (i.e., skill deficit and related components of the suicidal belief system). Not only does this improve understanding of the problem, but it also facilitates hope for recovery and improvement. Rather than the patient thinking about *10–15 episodes over the last 5 years*, he or she can identify two or three skill deficits responsible for every attempt. In helping make the problem more concrete, the clinician makes it more understandable and, ultimately, enhances the patient's hope for recovery and motivation for change. For example:

> "From the background we've talked about so far, it looks like this has been somewhat of a pattern over the years. You told me that you've made twelve attempts over the last six years. Have you noticed a pattern? Could you tell me what you've recognized that is similar across all of the suicide attempts you've made? If agreeable, I'd like to summarize the pattern that I see, at least from what you've told me so far. I may not be right in some of my assumptions but, if we put our heads together, I think we can probably come up

with a good model to explain what's been happening over the last six years."

4. Identify and explore the disadvantages of the deficit(s) (e.g., emotionally, physically, interpersonally, financially, and self-image) in order to enhance motivation for change and treatment.

> "It sounds like that over the years, your difficulty controlling anger and impulsivity have, in some ways, created even more problems for you. Does this sound accurate? Let's take, for example, the problem you voiced with anger management. What kinds of trouble has this created over the years?"

This can be followed with a specific discussion of emotional, physical, interpersonal, financial, and self-image consequences. For example, "I think you mentioned that the last time you got mad at work and impulsively said something to your supervisor you ended up getting fired, with financial problems shortly thereafter [interpersonal and financial consequences]. You also mentioned that, as a result of the difficult financial struggles you and your wife had to contend with that you ended up separating for a short period [interpersonal consequence]. Finally, I think you told me that this triggered your last episode of depression and you got highly critical and punitive toward yourself [emotional, self-image consequences]."

For the most part, we have found that if patients have an accurate understanding of the importance of targeting skill development in treatment, they are more than eager to comply. More often than not, clinicians that encounter resistance in this area have not fully explained where skill development *fits* in the treatment model. For the CBT approach described here, it is critical. As mentioned previously, cognitive restructuring of the suicidal belief system and skill building go hand in hand. For the most part, skill building is simply a series of *behavioral experiments,* each providing an opportunity for the patient to *draw a conclusion* and restructure a component of the suicidal belief system (even if specific to a single situation or circumstance). Actually, we have found that this is the component of treatment that patients enjoy the most, find easiest to understand, and frequently recall as *the most useful* in interviews at the end of treatment or during follow-up. When asking patients the question, "What did you find the most helpful during treatment?" responses such as being "taught how to be assertive and handle my anger," are relatively routine. At least from our experience, ensuring that the patient is adequately motivated amounts to ensuring that the patient is adequately informed.

Some Organizational Tasks for the Clinician to Remember across All Skill Areas

With respect to skill building, there are three general tasks for the clinician to remember. Although these tasks are essentially organizational in nature, they should not be dismissed as having limited value. Given the breadth of skills that will be targeted, the only way to ensure effective and efficient treatment is by imposing some general organizational guidelines. First, the clinician must determine what deficits are present. This is one of the identified goals of the initial interview(s), but will likely take a number of sessions (frequently two to three) to accomplish. Actually, the assessment of skill deficits is a continuous task throughout the entirety of treatment. It is likely, and probable, that the more meaningful deficits may not be identified until treatment has progressed. Often, underlying deficits are cloaked in the shroud of crisis symptoms, particularly with respect to interpersonal skills. Patients simply relate differently during periods of acute crisis and decompensation. For example, the clinician may find that the once passive and subjugated patient has *suddenly* become aggressive and hostile after a crisis has resolved, providing an important hint of previously unforeseen problems.

After identifying specific deficits, the clinician needs to consistently integrate skill training into the sessions in some format. Although this may sound easy, it can be difficult at times, particularly given that the key word here is "consistently." This integration can occur in many different ways, but perhaps the easiest is simply to make it a specific agenda item each and every session, allocating a predetermined amount of time. For example, 25 to 50% of each session (i.e., 15–30 minutes) could be spent targeting identified skill deficits. Also, the entire session(s) could be devoted to skill building, parceling off time to different content areas if desired. For example, 20 minutes could be devoted to anger management, 20 minutes to distress tolerance, and 20 minutes to interpersonal assertiveness. Similarly, a series of sessions could be devoted solely to skill building (e.g., sessions 5–10), depending on the needs of the patient, the progress of treatment, and time available.

Regardless of time devoted or the format introduced, it is important to ensure that the patient has an adequate understanding of the role played by a specific skill deficit when it is targeted in a session. As summarized previously, when reviewing the suicidal cycle with the patient and identifying specific points for intervention and treatment, skill building is one of the target areas discussed. It can be easily integrated into the conceptual discussion and the agenda simultaneously established for the session. For example:

THERAPIST: If you look at the cycle that we outlined, it looks like when you
    get acutely depressed, upset, and angry, you have trouble expressing the

anger in a way that you feel appropriate and healthy for you. Does this sound accurate?

PATIENT: That sounds about right. I get really mad and lose control.

THERAPIST: Then it looks like one of the things that we need to target for treatment is anger management, that is, let's help you deal with your anger in a more constructive way. Do you want to put that on the agenda today? It doesn't need to be the only thing we discuss but it does sound as though it's one of the more important problems you've experienced. Since there are a few other things that we need to talk about, what would you say if we devoted 20 minutes to anger management today?

The third and final point is that the clinician needs to periodically review the patient's identified skill deficits. The primary goal of the review is to update those that have been addressed, identify what stage of development the patient is demonstrating across each (i.e., as noted in Chapter 3, skill acquisition, skill refinement, or skill generalization), and target accordingly. It is easiest to use a hierarchy, as illustrated in Figure 10.1. The hierarchy concisely and effectively conveys which skill deficits are being targeted, which ones are most important and need to be targeted first, and what stage of development the patient is demonstrating for each. This can be kept as a part of the clinical record and amended or updated as needed. It is useful to periodically review the hierarchy with the patient to ensure agreement as to the treatment agenda.

As most clinicians are aware, the constraints on time-limited treatment are many. Accordingly, skill-building work needs to follow the same fundamental rules mentioned earlier for crisis intervention and cognitive restructuring. The general model employed needs to be *specific, simple*, and *accessible*. As a result, the skill-building modules covered in this chapter are relatively brief and straightforward, in both content and application. A basic model is provided for each, along with a discussion of applicable content and a few pointers about the process of implementation.

Each module can be expanded, deleted, or modified in accordance with clinical needs, theoretical approach, and time available. However, it is important to emphasize that each module has an *identifiable goal* deemed critical for treatment. The goal for each is provided here. If modifications are made, the clinician needs to be sure that this goal is still accomplished. Moreover, the clinician may find that we have not included enough topic areas and may want to expand the coverage provided. If so, it is important to remember the guideline referenced previously: The material needs to be specific, simple, and accessible. It should fit within the general framework of the suicidal mode, providing a means to identify, articulate, and modify components of the suicidal belief system.

Skill hierarchy: *Mr. G*

1. **Distress tolerance.** *The patient demonstrates poor distress tolerance. He has acted impulsively on his suicidal thoughts on several occasions. In addition, the patient's impulsivity is compounded by episodic alcohol abuse during periods of acute emotional upset. He also reports impulsivity in other areas of his life, stating that he frequently gets in arguments at work and home "without thinking" and on several occasions has gotten "physical" with his wife.* Skill acquisition.

2. **Self-monitoring.** *The patient demonstrates limited ability to self-monitor. He reports limited emotional awareness, has a difficult time identifying specific feelings and thoughts and has engaged in suicidal acts stating that "I don't know how I got there."* Some skill acquisition but predominantly skill refinement.

3. **Emotion regulation.** *The patient demonstrates poor emotion regulation ability, particularly at times of crisis. He reports that during periods of acute emotional upset and stress that he "stops doing things that help him feel better." He does demonstrate good emotion regulation ability during periods when he is not acutely stressed, reporting that he routinely exercises, spends time with his family, has a number of hobbies, and is very active in several social organizations.* Skill refinement and generalization.

4. **Anger management.** *The patient demonstrates some problems with anger. He reported on several occasions being motivated by anger when conflicts with his wife escalated to "physical confrontations." He also noted episodic anger at work, resulting in some verbal expression.* Some skill acquisition but predominantly skill refinement.

5. **Problem solving.** *The patient demonstrates limited ability to problem solve. He reports at times being easily overwhelmed. During his most recent suicidal crisis, he noted difficulty identifying the specific problem or generating alternative solutions.* Skill acquisition.

6. **Interpersonal skills.** *The patient demonstrates some problems in interpersonal skills, primarily revolving around assertiveness. He reported a style consistent with passivity and subjugation at times of conflict, often resulting in unexpressed anger.* Skill acquisition.

FIGURE 10.1. Example of a skill deficit hierarchy.

It is also important to note that the role of group treatment is discussed in detail in Chapter 3. Many of the modules are greatly enhanced by the use of a group format for this component of treatment, despite the fact that much of the material will undoubtedly be covered in individual sessions as well. The use of a group format for skill training has innumerable benefits, which are reviewed in Chapter 3. Actually, in our treatment program we have found that problem-solving training and interpersonal skills are most effectively taught in a group setting, particularly given the importance of role playing and behavioral rehearsal. Many clinicians, however, do not have this option. The modules provided can easily be covered in individual or group format. Ideally, patients would have access to both, with skill building done in a group setting, serving as a powerful complement to ongoing individual treatment. The interpersonal context provides a mechanism to *activate* the *other* component (i.e., beliefs that others are rejecting, abusing, abandoning, and judgmental) of the suicidal belief system that, at times, may appear dormant in individual sessions. Individual sessions can be used to reinforce, expand, tailor, or simply repeat material covered in the group sessions. In short, if the clinician has group format available, it can serve as a powerful and meaningful complement to individual work, due primarily to the very nature of the suicidal belief system described.

A Model for Problem Solving: Learning to Identify, Evaluate, and Pursue Alternatives to Suicide

Primary goal: To teach the patient to effectively problem-solve by eliminating extreme (and impulsive) responding and avoidance, developing a structured and methodical approach, and acquiring the skills necessary for flexible living (e.g., assertiveness and emotion regulation).

For the suicidal patient, problem-solving deficits are often numerous and varied. The patient may have difficulty simply defining the problem at hand, delaying an impulsive reaction, generating realistic alternatives, effectively evaluating those alternatives (over both the short and the long term), implementing a decision, and evaluating its efficacy in order to determine future actions. Given the broad range of possibilities, we recommend the use of a structured and methodical approach to problem solving. We have adapted and somewhat modified the sequential approach of Nezu et al.(1989).

Six sequential steps are recommended:

1. Define the problem.
2. Identify your goal.
3. Generate alternatives.

4. Evaluate the alternatives.
5. Implement one.
6. Evaluate your initial efforts and modify your approach.

We have found it most effective to implement, and consistently make use of, a structured approach. It is easiest to put the problem-solving steps on a *coping card* (see Figure 10.2), provide it to the patient, and use it every time a specific problem is addressed. The coping card can be carried in a wallet or purse or as a part of the patient's treatment log. The coping card provides a series of prompt questions to guide the patient through the process. This approach can be applied to a broad range of problems, including interpersonal conflicts, financial troubles, and physical illness, among a host of others. Although it is recommended that problem solving be introduced early in the treatment process, it is important to remember that it needs to be done *consistently* and *methodically* over the entirety of treatment, not just covered during one or two sessions and then never mentioned again. For example, the following exchange illustrates how problem solving can be integrated in a relatively seamless fashion regardless of the topic.

PATIENT: I've been feeling pretty great the last two weeks. I hadn't thought about suicide one time. Then, yesterday, my boss comes in and tells me what a sorry job I did handling a call last week. Somebody complained and he came in and just let me have it! I really got down, later in the day I just thought, "What's the use in trying? I fail anyway." Then I thought about killing myself. I wasn't really serious, but the idea just flashed through my head.

THERAPIST: This might be a good time to review some of what we talked about last month about problem solving. Do you have your coping card with you? Let's plug in this problem and go through it. Maybe we can figure out where you ran into trouble and why those thoughts about suicide surfaced. You've had some success in problem solving lately but I wonder if you really believe in your skills?

Problem-solving training can be greatly enhanced by the use of both large and small groups, an issue discussed in detail in the Chapter 3. In addition, videotaping and audiotaping sessions is extremely valuable. We have found that patients respond quite well to the routine audiotaping of sessions, which allows them the opportunity to review the session both at their leisure and repeatedly if needed. Periodic videotaping of sessions, for review with the patient in subsequent meetings, can be invaluable in helping the patient identify and review strengths and weaknesses. Videotaping can supplement the problem-solving process, complementing behavioral rehearsal and role play-

1. **Define the problem.** Summarize the problem in one sentence. If there is more than one problem, pick the one that is most important **right now.** If you believe the problem is too big, break it into three identifiable parts. Put them in the order necessary to solve it.

2. **Identify your goal.** Write down your goal. What do you hope to accomplish in the immediate future? Over the long run? If you can't identify a goal, you've likely not defined the problem well. Go back and restate it and try again.

3. **Generate alternatives.** How many alternatives can you identify? Remember to suspend judgment at this point. Simply identify as many options as you can. If you're having trouble, consider discussing the problem with significant others or those who have previously demonstrated responsibility in your relationship.

4. **Evaluate the alternatives.** Now it is time to evaluate the alternatives. Ask yourself the following questions. Can I realistically do what I've identified? What is required in order to implement the option I've selected? How much time, energy, and effort? Is it consistent with my values? What will be the effects on myself, family, and friends right now and down the road?

5. **Implement one.** Select the best alternative and implement it. Ask yourself a few simple questions. What steps are necessary to implement the option selected? Is it something you can do alone, or do you need the assistance of someone else?

6. **Evaluate your initial efforts and modify your approach.** How did things turn out? Did it work? If not, what went wrong? What can you learn from this initial effort (if it was unsuccessful) in order to try again? If you've learned something, go back to Step 4 and try again. If not, start at Step 1. Regardless of the outcome, remember two things. First, you're actively trying to solve a difficult problem. And second, you're not acting impulsively.

FIGURE 10.2. Problem-solving coping card. From *Treating Suicidal Behavior: An Effective, Time-Limited Approach* by M. David Rudd, Thomas Joiner, and M. Hasan Rajab. Copyright 2001 by The Guilford Press. Permission to reproduce this figure is granted to purchasers of this book for personal use only (see copyright page for details).

ing where and when appropriate. It is also an excellent way to monitor treatment progress over time. There is nothing quite as powerful as a videotaped session to help the patient see, in very concrete terms, the progress he or she has made over a few months.

Emotion Regulation Ability: The Art of *Feeling Better* When Suicidal

Primary goal: To help the patient identify, express, and respond more effectively (i.e., shorten recovery time) to emotions experienced when acutely stressed and suicidal.

Emotion regulation can be defined simply as the *ability to identify, understand, express, and respond effectively to the full range of human emotions.* Many suicidal patients express discomfort with not only their own emotional needs but also affective experience in general. As illustrated with the case of Mr. G discussed previously, he had trouble identifying specific feelings, expressing them in a constructive manner, and then taking steps that would help him more effectively regulate the emotional experience, particularly over the short term (e.g., going out and exercising rather than going to the bar when acutely depressed). Suicidal patients present with emotion regulation problems that cut across the full spectrum ranging from problems with identification (i.e., emotional awareness and acceptance) and expression (i.e., either constriction or excessive lability) to response (i.e., behaviors that facilitate recovery rather than intensification of the negative emotion). Accordingly, the goal is pretty simple and straightforward: Help the patient identify the feeling, express it appropriately, and respond in a manner that reduces observed and experienced suicidality.

As with all the skill-building modules, we recommend a simple approach, one that the patient can retain and use daily. As with the problem-solving module, a coping card can be used but often is not necessary given the relative simplicity of the approach recommended. The patient should be taught the following three steps:

1. *Identify* the feeling. Label the feeling. Answer the question "How do you feel?" *Not* "What do you think?" See how much you can broaden the range of feelings you recognize and experience over time. Make an effort to become more precise about your feelings as treatment progresses. If you're struggling to identify the feeling, ask yourself, "How would someone else feel if he or she were in my shoes?" Also, if you can't identify the feeling, what do you notice physically? Are there physical sensations consistent with any par-

ticular feeling (e.g., clinching your fist when angry, pacing and physical tension when anxious, agitated, or apprehensive)?

2. *Express* what you feel in some way. Go beyond just labeling your feeling(s). You might want to write about it in your journal, draw a picture, or find another method of expression (e.g., a poem). Try not to restrict what you feel, but make an effort to be spontaneous (and appropriate) in your expressions. Find methods of expression that you feel good about. When you've successfully tried them, make note and keep a list in your treatment journal.

3. *Respond* so as to facilitate your recovery. Do something to facilitate recovery from negative feelings (e.g., sadness, anger, frustration, irritation, shame, and guilt). This more than likely will mean changing some of the self-defeating and destructive behaviors you've identified earlier. If you can't identify something that will help you feel better, don't do anything that can make you feel worse (e.g., drinking, isolating yourself or withdrawing). You can always do an STR! Review your crisis coping card for steps that you can take to facilitate your recovery (e.g., taking a walk, talking to a good friend, taking a hot bath, listening to music, reading your treatment log, reading a book). In short, what can you do to help yourself feel better? If some problem solving is required first, review your problem-solving coping card and follow the steps listed.

Emotion regulation is a skill that needs to be integrated, in some capacity, into every session. As mentioned previously, emotion regulation is one of the three *core interventions*. For the most part, emotion regulation will be inherent to almost every aspect of the treatment agenda. This can be accomplished in a simple manner. The clinician simply needs to articulate specifically for the patient when *effective* (and similarly *ineffective*) emotion regulation is accomplished. This is facilitated by use of the subjective ratings referenced previously for risk assessment (i.e., using rating scales of 1 to 10 for feelings and symptoms). The specific steps taken, or techniques used, for effective emotion regulation can then be identified, discussed, and added to the patient's crisis response plan and related coping card(s). For example:

THERAPIST: When we started today, you mentioned that you were very angry. Actually, I think you rated it as a 9. How do you feel now?

PATIENT: Well, I guess it's about a 5 or 6 now.

THERAPIST: That seems like a pretty substantial change in a relatively short period of time. I think that is particularly important since you originally told me that you believed that your "feelings never change quickly when you're angry" and also that you believed there "was nothing you could do to feel better." What exactly did we do to facilitate your recovery, that is, help your anger dissipate?

PATIENT: I don't know, what did we do? It seems like all we did was talk.

THERAPIST: You're right, we didn't have to do that much. Basically, two things happened. First, time passed, actually only thirty minutes or so. Second, we talked and you were provided with an outlet for your anger. You expressed it in an appropriate and healthy way. Can you come to any conclusions about how you handle your anger?

PATIENT: Well, I guess I can conclude that if I just talk about my feelings and wait a little while, the anger will go away, at least enough that I don't blow up.

THERAPIST: Sounds like an important conclusion to come to!

To a large degree, emotion regulation will involve cognitive restructuring (as referenced earlier). The patient will likely hold specific beliefs about particular feelings. Often, the most problematic beliefs will revolve around negative affect, such as sadness, frustration, anger, shame, or guilt (among others). It is important to integrate cognitive restructuring into the process when appropriate. This is relatively easy to do; simply help the patient recognize *affect shifts* during sessions, articulate previously stated (and relevant) intermediate and core beliefs, and offer the opportunity for new conclusions (i.e., new core beliefs).

The majority of these beliefs will revolve around the *self-component* (e.g., "I'll never stop feeling this way") of the suicidal belief system. However, beliefs about *others* ("I only hurt people I care about when I get mad") and the *future* ("I'll never get better at doing this") will also apply. It will be important to keep tabs and monitor these new beliefs over time, essentially compiling evidence to support them over the course of treatment. It is perhaps most efficient, not to mention effective, to have patients keep a record of changing core beliefs as a part of their treatment log and belief hierarchy, mentioned in Chapter 9.

Self-Monitoring

Primary goal: To help the patient improve his or her overall awareness, insight, understanding, and acceptance of natural emotional fluctuations in day-to-day living.

Self-monitoring refers to the simple task of having patients monitor what they are thinking, feeling, and doing. Much of this was covered in Chapters 6 and 7 but bear repeating here. Clearly, self-monitoring and emotion regulation are interdependent. To respond more effectively to negative affect changes, the patient must first be aware that a change has actually occurred. As mentioned earlier, self-monitoring needs to be implemented immediately and continued in some way throughout the entirety of treatment. In many ways, the simple act of implementing self-monitoring reduces impulsivity. Consistent with the notion of *purposeful hypervigilance* presented earlier, the patient's heightened focus and awareness is incompatible with impulsive behavior, essentially consistent with the concept of reciprocal inhibition.

There are a number of ways to facilitate the development of self-monitoring skills, among the easiest and most direct are:

- Use of the STR on a regular basis.
- Use of recurrent subjective ratings for feelings and symptoms.
- Repeated drawings, and appropriate modifications, of the patient's suicidal cycle.
- Consistent use of the treatment log or daily journal.
- Use of a daily, weekly, or monthly mood graph targeting a specific, problem emotion (e.g., shame, guilt, and anger).
- Use of audio or videotaping, specifically for later review and analysis in session.

Regardless of the method chosen, self-monitoring can be presented and reviewed in fairly simple terms for the patient. The general idea is to promote emotional awareness, understanding (i.e., acceptance), and more effective responding (see Chapter 3). As with the other skills reviewed in this chapter, self-monitoring can also be summarized on a coping card which the patient can carry. If the process of developing multiple coping cards becomes too cumbersome, the patient can develop a single card with multiple skills summarized (i.e., a skill-building card). Actually, it might be easiest to combine the emotion regulation and self-monitoring cards. As noted later, the last step instructs the patient to implement his or her emotion regulation plan. The self-monitoring card should include, at a minimum, the following three steps:

1. *Label* what you are feeling. If it is more than one feeling, try to be precise. List all feelings that you recognize.
2. *Understand* your feelings. Recognize and accept that feelings are *normal*. There is a reason you are having the feeling(s). Although the feeling may be disproportionate for any number of reasons (e.g., your personal history, recent stressor), it is not wrong. Letting it go unchecked can create problems though. Remember, you can influence the intensity of the feeling and how long it might last.
3. *Respond* to more effectively regulate the feeling(s). Implement your emotion regulation skills (i.e., express the feelings appropriately and take steps to facilitate recovery) and reevaluate things in a few minutes.

Distress Tolerance

Primary goal: To help the patient improve his or her ability to tolerate negative emotions (i.e., to be less reactive and impulsive), raise his or her threshold for initial activation, diffuse rapid onset of emotional upset, and shorten the time required for recovery.

As is evident, self-monitoring, emotion regulation, and distress tolerance are all interdependent. In particular, the latter two are dependent on the first. In some ways, poor distress tolerance prevents effective emotion regulation. Similarly, distress tolerance and impulsivity are interdependent constructs. In short, patients who demonstrate poor distress tolerance have a tendency to act impulsively. As Linehan (1993) has so aptly noted, suicidal patients (particularly chronically suicidal patients) tend to demonstrate high reactivity in terms of both a low threshold for activation and rapid onset of emotional upset. They also tend to evidence more severe reactions and longer recovery periods, something often confounded by difficulty with emotion regulation (i.e., they tend to *do things* that intensify rather than diffuse the emotional response). Actually, some of our findings have confirmed more severe and complex emotional symptoms among multiple attempters (Rudd, Joiner, & Rajab, 1996).

As with self-monitoring and emotion regulation, distress tolerance is addressed during every session (most prominently during periods of acute crisis), regardless of whether the patient or clinician acknowledges it. Distress tolerance will naturally parallel self-monitoring and emotion regulation development. It is important, however, for the clinician to be aware of several issues and work diligently to emphasize the importance of this skill throughout the entirety of treatment.

- Consistent with the theory underlying exposure-based (CBT) treatments, distress tolerance should improve both across and within sessions, that is, if self-monitoring and emotion regulation skills improve. To monitor progress, the clinician needs to be aware of, and to review with the patient, the characteristics summarized earlier. This can be done simply by reviewing the patient's relative threshold for emotional upset (i.e., *how much it took to get the patient upset*), reactivity (i.e., *speed and severity of upset*), and time required for recovery (i.e., it should shorten over time, possibly for multiple episodes of emotional upset during a single session). For example:

> "I just want to point out that today, when you got upset at your wife, it sounded as though it took a lot longer before you got upset, it wasn't as severe, and you recovered much quicker. Does that sound accurate? What does that tell you, is there anything you can conclude about your distress tolerance ability?"

[later in the same session] "You know, you got upset on three different occasions today when we discussed that fight with your wife. Each time, you appeared to be less upset and you recovered more quickly. Did you notice that as well?"

• Distress tolerance can be purposefully tested by periodically (and strategically) reviewing particularly *hot topics*, that is, those with strong developmental relevance and potency (e.g., physical, sexual, and emotional abuse during childhood and adolescence) for the patient. This should, however, be discussed and coordinated with the patient and pursued in a cautious and conservative fashion. This is likely most important for patients evidencing chronic suicidal behavior.

Interpersonal Skills: Learning to Be Assertive, Attentive, and Responsive

Primary goal: To help the patient improve his or her interpersonal awareness, comfort, and skills (i.e., assertiveness, attentiveness, and responsiveness).

Given the broad range of interpersonal skills that can potentially be taught, we recommend focusing on a few that are consistently found to be problematic, all revolving around issues of interpersonal assertiveness. We recommend targeting three areas: interpersonal assertiveness, attentiveness, and responsiveness. Focusing on attentiveness and responsiveness as well as assertiveness helps the patient become more aware of the highly interactive and interdependent nature of a social interaction.

Many suicidal patients experience considerable difficulty with passivity, avoidance, and subjugation. Given issues of chronicity, interpersonal assertiveness can be one of the most difficult skills to target, frequently requiring some form of group format for effective change. As with the other skill areas covered, it is easiest to develop a coping card addressing the general topic of interpersonal skills. The following format is only one possibility:

• *Assertiveness* (voicing your thoughts, feelings, and needs in an appropriate way). Practice voicing your thoughts, feelings, and needs in an open, appropriate, and non-aggressive manner. Try to monitor the tone of your voice, rate and rhythm of your speech, your facial expression (e.g., Are you smiling?) and behavior (e.g., posture, Are you making eye contact? What are you doing with your hands? How far are you standing from the person to whom you're talking?). Do you have more trouble with certain people? If so, do you notice doing anything different? What thoughts do you notice going through your head at those times?

- *Attentiveness* (listening to the thoughts, feelings, and needs of others). Practice attending to what others are saying. Follow up with a question based on what was said to you to make sure you understand what is being said (i.e., clarify the conversation or interaction).
- *Responsiveness* (responding to the requests of others). Practice responding to the requests of others. Model the behavior that you'd like others to demonstrate. If you disagree with someone about a particular issue, particularly one that you feel very strongly about, can you stop things from escalating? Is there something about their position you can agree with?

As with all the skills referenced, it is critical to concurrently target cognitive restructuring, identifying and articulating specifically the automatic thoughts and intermediate and core beliefs that comprise interpersonal aspects of the suicidal belief system (i.e., beliefs about *others*). Some of the most salient beliefs revolve around interactions with others. This is perhaps the area in which videotaping of role plays and related behavioral rehearsal exercises is most effective. Videotape (and audiotape if it is the only option available) can assist the patient in recognizing things about his or her interpersonal style that previously had gone unnoticed. It provides an opportunity to break interactions down into details with respect to tone of voice, rate and rhythm of speech, posture, hand gestures, eye contact, and personal space, among a host of others. Actually, interpersonal skills are most effectively taught in a group context.

Anger Management: Early Identification, Appropriate Expression, and the Importance of Empathy, Acceptance, and Forgiveness

Primary goal: To help the patient improve his or her ability to recognize the early signs of anger, identify whether or not the anger is appropriate and proportional to the trigger, intervene early, and express it in a constructive and healthy manner. In addition, it is important for the patient to recognize that empathy, acceptance, and forgiveness are all essential to dealing effectively with anger.

Anger management training has three primary targets. The first is to help the patient become more aware of early markers of significant anger. Such markers cut across each domain of daily functioning, including cognitive, emotional/physiological (physical sensations), and behavioral. Day-to-day self-monitoring using the suicidal cycle and the STR are the easiest and most efficient ways to identify early markers. Once identified, steps can be taken to address and diffuse the patient's anger early in the cycle (consistent with the previous discussion of reducing and eliminating suicidal behavior). The goal is to prevent rapid and uncontrollable escalation, primarily as a function of increasing the amount of time available for intervention. As the amount of time available for intervention increases, so does opportunity, in terms of both the frequency of intervention efforts and the duration of those attempted.

Again, the use of an anger coping card is recommended. A general card can be used, cutting across any anger-provoking situation, or a specific one can be developed that targets a particularly problematic situation or circumstance (see Figure 10.3). As illustrated in Figure 10.3, the steps recommended need to be simple and straightforward. A complicated series of steps during periods of acute anger are simply unreasonable and may only increase frustration, further escalating the problem. In many ways, an anger coping card is simply a situation-specific emotion regulation exercise. Nonetheless, given its prominence among suicidal patients as a specifically identified problem or complaint, it is important to address anger in a focused and detailed manner. The primary goal of the anger coping card is to facilitate early intervention, diffusing potential escalation and impulsive, self-defeating, or self-destructive behavior. If acute-onset anger is a particular problem for the patient, it will probably be necessary to make use of role playing and practice with the coping card. Videotaping is extremely valuable under these circumstances.

In addition to early recognition and intervention, it is important not only to help the patient develop an understanding of appropriate anger expression but also to provide a consistent and accessible outlet. Role playing (in conjunction with assertiveness training) is an effective tool but one greatly facilitated by the development and use of an *anger log*. We encourage patients to keep an anger log, which simply amounts to an anger hierarchy or list. They can simply transfer anger precipitating events, circumstances, or other issues from their STR or daily treatment journal. Once the hierarchy is developed, each event, circumstance, or issue can be targeted individually and strategically. Often, little more is required than an opportunity for the patient to ventilate. However, it is sometimes necessary to plug each issue identified as warranting further attention into the problem-solving model summarized earlier in order to identify a specific plan of action that might provide relief. Once again, this problem-solving process is greatly enhanced by the use of role playing, behavioral rehearsal, and videotaping.

We believe it is important for suicidal patients to ask a few cogent questions about their anger before deciding whether to apply the problem-solving model referenced earlier. In many ways, the series of questions proposed amounts to cognitive restructuring. Without answering these questions, the anger is often so poorly understood that pursuing problem solving is simply pointless. As with other skills covered here, these steps (and questions) can

Step 1. Stop and recognize what you're angry about. What are you thinking? What do you notice physically? Rate your anger on a scale of 1–10.

Step 2. Ask yourself the following question, is it worth doing anything about right now? Does it really matter? How important will this be in a few hours, tomorrow?

Step 3. If it is an important issue and warrants a response, implement your problem-solving coping card, make a decision about your alternatives, and do something identified as appropriate.

Step 4. If it isn't important and won't matter in a few hours or tomorrow, then take a few minutes to recover. Leave the situation if needed. Stop and count to 20, say the alphabet backwards. Do an imagery or relaxation exercise. Rate your anger again; repeat until your anger drops to a 7 or below.

FIGURE 10.3. Anger coping card. From *Treating Suicidal Behavior: An Effective, Time-Limited Approach* by M. David Rudd, Thomas Joiner, and M. Hasan Rajab. Copyright 2001 by The Guilford Press. Permission to reproduce this figure is granted to purchasers of this book for personal use only (see copyright page for details).

also be put on a coping card to facilitate learning. More than likely, though, this series of questions will need to be addressed repeatedly throughout the entirety of treatment. Consistent with the goal of *building more adaptive modes*, an effort is being made to help the patient *think differently* about experienced anger. Accordingly, a few of the intermediate and core beliefs comprising the suicidal belief system will need to be specifically identified and targeted. Among the proposed questions are the following:

1. "What exactly are you angry about? Try to summarize it in one sentence. If you can't, try to identify more than one thing that you're angry about. Describe each in a sentence."
2. "What triggered your anger? Was it one thing, or an accumulation of things over time?"
3. "Is your anger proportionate or appropriate to what triggered it? Does it seem too intense? For example, if someone cut you off on the highway, are you enraged and ready to run him or her off the road? If your anger is proportionate and appropriate, can you problem solve and respond in an appropriate way?"
4. "If your anger is disproportionate (i.e., too intense), what do you think the problem is? Distinguish whether or not it's *old* anger. Old anger is anger that's been around and accumulating for a period of time, anywhere from a few hours to early in the day to years. Often times, it's compounded by childhood and developmental problems such as early emotional wounds of some sort (physical, sexual, emotional abuse). Did someone just trigger old anger? Did something happen earlier in the day that your angry about, something last week, last month, last year? Did somebody push one of your buttons about things that happened when you were younger that have never been adequately resolved?"
5. "If it is old anger, is there really anything you can do about it? If not, then work on acceptance, empathy, and forgiveness."
6. Can you come to some conclusion about your anger in this specific situation or circumstance? Write down your conclusion in your treatment log or journal.

As evidenced in the foregoing series of questions, acceptance, empathy and forgiveness are often the only effective means of addressing chronic anger. They can be approached from many different perspectives, depending in part on the spiritual and religious orientation of the patient, as well as the theoretical orientation of the clinician. It is important for clinician and patient to come to some agreement as to how these constructs *fit into* their conceptualization of anger, particularly chronic anger. As noted previously, attentiveness and responsiveness are addressed as part of interpersonal skills. This provides an opening for targeting empathy and forgiveness as interventions for both chronic and acute anger, depending on the circumstances. Regardless of the clinician's approach to acceptance, empathy, and forgiveness, it is important to emphasize that although these are relatively abstract concepts for each to be achieved it *must* be demonstrated. That is, it must be evident in the individual's behavior and manner of relating. Consistent with the CBT framework proposed, the clinician should identify and articulate each component system of the new adaptive mode in order to confirm the presence of acceptance, empathy, or forgiveness. In short, if any of these are accomplished, the patient will be thinking, feeling, and behaving differently.

Skill Building and Personality Change: One and the Same?

Personality disorders are defined in DSM-IV (American Psychiatric Association, 1994) as pervasive, inflexible patterns of behavior that create distress and dysfunction in social and/or occupational arenas. By definition, then, skill building is essentially comparable to personality change. If patients are successful in developing, refining, and generalizing skills, they have, by definition, evidenced personality change. This is particularly true if skill building concurrently targets related automatic thoughts, conditional rules and assumptions (intermediate beliefs), and core beliefs. Actually, it would be difficult *not* to effect change in the patient's suicidal belief system if change occurred in his or her day-to-day skills. Given the interdependent and interactive nature of the component systems of the suicidal mode, effective skill building is, in essence, the process of establishing more adaptive modes for the suicidal patient. As each targeted skill generalizes, the new adaptive mode becomes more accessible and meaningful for the patient. In short, the Axis II pathology noted begins to show signs of resolving.

Changing Interpersonal Process: Integrating Group Treatment

In recognition of the critical role played by interpersonal relationships in any explanatory model of suicidality, it is desirable that treatment, at a minimum, attempt to incorporate some group component if at all possible. Naturally, there will be circumstances or situations, driven by many factors, that make this impossible. The treatment model we offer is very much amenable to either a group component or complement in some form or fashion. Actually, in our original outcome study, all the problem-solving training was provided in a group context, incorporating both large and small groups (Rudd, Rajab, et al., 1996). In terms of the treatment model provided, there are essentially four group options: (1) psychoeducational groups, (2) large problem-solving groups, (3) small problem-solving groups, and (4) interpersonal process groups. These are discussed in more detail later. As mentioned in Chapter 3, interpersonal process groups can be helpful in the role of booster sessions *after* individual treatment.

The advantages of incorporating a group component into treatment are varied. First and foremost, integrating a group component provides a unique opportunity to directly target the interpersonal factors that are, in all likelihood, implicated in the patient's suicidality. Second, it offers a chance to directly address and practice the coping skills that are vital to successful treatment, ideally leading to more effective and lasting change. Third, it offers a chance to provide some uniformity and consistency in treatment across providers in a particular setting, addressing to some degree the issue of treatment fidelity. Fourth, for those with limited resources and time, it is probably the most efficient treatment mechanism. Fifth, it diffuses treatment responsibilities into a treatment *team*, incorporating multiple clinicians into the treatment process. This is particularly important for those treating suicidality on a consistent basis. Everyone needs support, clinicians included. As a result of using common groups for some of the purposes summarized previously, there is a need for treatment team meetings to address coordination of care, successes, and conflicts, among a host of other issues. In short, integration of a group component to treatment has many important advantages, only one of which is effective and efficient care.

Psychoeducational Groups

Psychoeducational groups can be used to complement a patient's ongoing individual therapy, particularly in a setting in which resources are limited and time constraints severe. The recommended format, and the one that we have used, is to implement a primary psychoeducational group that meets concurrently with individual therapy for a limited period of time, say for 5 to 8 sessions over a period of 2 to 4 months. The group is used for basic education regarding the skills training discussed earlier in this chapter and includes patients from all providers actively treating suicidality. The material provided earlier can easily be translated into curriculum format, one session for each content area (i.e., problem solving, emotion regulation, self-monitoring, distress tolerance, interpersonal skills, and anger management). Additional sessions can be developed and included covering topics such as cognitive restructuring, crisis management, and developmental trauma, depending on the clinician's particular needs or setting.

To use psychoeducational groups efficiently and effectively, we recommend a number of general guidelines:

- Clearly define the purpose of the group for patients referred. Psychoeducational groups need to be fairly structured in format. The primary goal is to *cover a basic curriculum and convey specific content*, not to provide an opportunity for group exploration and discussion. If this expectation is clear from the very beginning, a considerable number of problems can be avoided.

- Operate the group as a closed group with a fixed and predictable schedule. The group can operate on a fixed, rotational schedule (e.g., once every quarter) that is predictable for both participating clinicians and patients. We have also found that psychoeducational groups operate best if they are relatively small (e.g., four to seven members). This provides an opportunity for some limited discussion, clarification of information provided, and related questions. A fixed schedule lets patients schedule their participation from the very beginning, making arrangements at home and/or work. In addition, the small size provides a chance for some cohesiveness to develop despite the educational goal and learning format of the group.

- Guard against the group evolving into a process group. This is easiest to do by being clear about the goal(s) when the group starts. As noted later, if a process group is needed, the clinician should develop and implement one specifically for this purpose. Occasionally, members will attempt to shift the focus of the group. This does not imply that group process should be inhibited; rather, it should be constrained within the context of a psychoeducational format. This can be done in many ways, but most effectively by limiting the duration of the group (e.g., 1 hour) and gentle reminders when necessary.

- Develop a specific curriculum outline for each session. The skills building covered earlier in the chapter easily translates into a curriculum format, as does much of what is covered in terms of cognitive restructuring and crisis intervention. Actually, much of this material is *already* in a curriculum format (e.g., specific steps for crisis management, problem solving, and anger management).

Problem-Solving Groups (Large and Small)

The use of problem-solving groups can be highly effective. In our program, we distinguished between large and small groups. We frequently had anywhere from 9 to 12 individuals in our large groups. These groups were closed and on a fixed, rotational schedule. For these groups to be effective, it is necessary to allocate larger blocks of time. Our groups routinely ran for 2 hours. The large group was used entirely for psychoeducational purposes. Specifically, the basic tenets of effective problem solving covered earlier were reviewed in detail (e.g., for 30 to 45 minutes). We would then separate into small groups (i.e., three to four members maximum), using multiple therapists, for problem-solving practice addressing specific problems generated by group members. In all cases, the problems targeted were those that precipitated the patients' suicidal crises. Often, the problems were taken directly from the patients' self-monitoring logs, treatment journals, or STRs.

The small groups followed a specific sequence. Each member would identify a specific problem and apply the problem-solving steps reviewed earlier, with assistance provided by the therapist and other group members. Once a preferable alternative was identified, it would be implemented and practiced by role play. If the role play revealed specific deficits, areas of weakness, or problems, those would be targeted in subsequent efforts. If an alternative did not appear effective, new alternatives were generated and practiced. In general, the small groups provided fertile ground to practice and refine possible solutions. Frequently these role plays were videotaped for review with the large group in later sessions, with subsequent critique and discussion. Criticism by other group members can be handled as a specific interpersonal problem for subsequent role plays. It is a great opportunity to practice problem solving with regard to the experience of receiving criticism. It is easiest and most effective to rotate videotaping among the small groups. For example, each week a different small group could be taped. Reviewing the tapes in the large group provides patients an opportunity to see *how others do it*. In addition, it provides a unique opportunity to identify and discuss common problem areas. Frequently, it is apparent that a particular set of skills (e.g., assertiveness) needs to be targeted in more depth by the small groups. As a result, changes can be made in terms of how time is allocated for large and small group activities.

All in all, we have found the large and small problem-solving groups to be a tremendous resource, well received by patients. They provide a truly unique opportunity to engage in interpersonal problem solving in a very active and realistic manner. The primary goal of problem-solving groups, large or small, is to help the patient actually *practice* interpersonal problem-solving skills. This, naturally, involves the application of other interpersonal skills. Accordingly, it is a rich intervention and one, we believe, central to lasting change.

References

Abramson, L. Y., Metalsky, G. I., & Alloy, L. B. (1989). Hopelessness depression: A theory-based subtype of depression. *Psychological Review, 96*(2), 358–372.

Alford, B. A., & Beck, A. T. (1997). *The integrative power of cognitive therapy.* New York: Guilford Press.

Allard, R., Marshall, M., & Plante, M. (1992). Intensive follow-up does not decrease the risk of repeat suicide attempts. *Suicide and Life-Threatening Behavior, 22,* 303–314.

American Psychiatric Association. (1994). *Diagnostic and statistical manual of mental disorders* (4th ed.). Washington, DC: Author.

Arnkoff, D. B., & Glass, C. R. (1992). Cognitive therapy and psychotherapy integration. In D. K. Freedheim (Ed.), *History of psychotherapy: A century of change* (pp. 657–694). Washington, DC: American Psychological Association.

Bandura, A. (1986). *Social foundations of thought and action: A social cognitive theory.* Englewood Cliffs, NJ: Prentice-Hall.

Barnett, J. (1998). Termination without trepidation. *Psychotherapy Bulletin, 33*(2), 20–22.

Battin, M. (1982). *Ethical issues in suicide.* Englewood Cliffs, NJ: Prentice-Hall.

Beck, A. T. (1964). Thinking and depression: II. Theory and therapy. *Archives of General Psychiatry, 10,* 561–571.

Beck, A. T. (1976). *Cognitive therapy and the emotional disorders.* New York: New American Library.

Beck, A. T. (1996). Beyond belief: A theory of modes, personality, and psychopathology (pp. 1–25). In P. Salkovskis (Ed.), *Frontiers of cognitive therapy.* New York: Guilford Press.

Beck, A. T., Brown, G., Berchick, R., & Stewart, B. (1990). Relationship between hopelessness and ultimate suicide: A replication with psychiatric outpatients. *American Journal of Psychiatry, 147,* 190–195.

Beck, A. T., Brown, G., Berchick, R. J., Stewart, B. L., & Steer, R. A. (1990). Relationships between hopelessness and ultimate suicide: A replication with psychiatric outpatients. *American Journal of Psychiatry, 147*(2), 190–195.

Beck, A. T., Emery, G., & Greenberg, R. L. (1985). *Anxiety disorders and phobias: A cognitive perspective.* New York: Basic Books.

Beck, A. T., Freeman, A., & Associates. (1990). *Cognitive therapy of personality disorders.* New York: Guilford Press.

Beck, A. T., & Lester, D. (1976). Components of suicide intent in attempted and completed suicide. *Journal of Psychology, 92,* 35–38.

Beck, A. T., Kovacs, M., & Weissman, A. (1975). Hopelessness and suicidal behavior: An overview. *Journal of the American Medical Association, 234*(11), 1146–1149.

Beck, A. T., Rush, A. J., Shaw, B. F., & Emery, G. (1979). *Cognitive therapy of depression.* New York: Guilford Press.

Beck, A. T., & Steer, R. A. (1988). *Beck Hopelessness Scale manual.* San Antonio: Psychological Corporation.

Beck, A. T., & Steer, R. A. (1993). *Beck Scale for Suicide Ideation manual.* San Antonio: Psychological Corporation.

Beck, A. T., Steer, R. A., & Brown, G. (1993). Dysfunctional attitudes and suicidal ideation in psychiatric outpatients. *Suicide and Life-Threatening Behavior, 23*(1), 11–20.

Beck, A. T., Steer, R. A., & Brown, G. (1996). *BDI—II manual.* San Antonio: Psychological Corporation.

Beck, J. S. (1995). *Cognitive therapy: Basics and beyond.* New York: Guilford Press.

Berman, A. L., & Jobes, D. A. (1991). *Adolescent suicide: Assessment and intervention.* Washington, DC: American Psychological Association.

Bongar, B. (Ed.). (1991). *The suicidal patient: Clinical and legal standards of care.* Washington, DC: American Psychological Association.

Bongar, B. (Ed.). (1992). *Suicide: Guidelines for assessment, management, and treatment.* New York: Oxford University Press.

Bongar, B., & Harmatz (1989). Graduate training in clinical psychology and the study of suicide. *Professional Psychology: Research and Practice, 20,* 209–213.

Bongar, B., Maris, R., Berman, A., & Litman, R. (1992). Outpatient standards of care and the suicidal patient. *Suicide and Life-Threatening Behavior, 22,* 453–478.

Bongar, B., Maris, R., Berman, A., Litman, R., & Silverman, M. (1993). Inpatient standards of care and the suicidal patient. Part I: General clinical formulations and legal considerations. *Suicide and Life-Threatening Behavior, 23,* 245–256.

Bongar, B., Peterson, L. G., Harris, E. A., & Aissis, J. (1989). Clinical and legal considerations in the management of suicidal patients: An integrative overview. *Journal of Integrative and Eclectic Psychotherapy, 8*(1), 53–67.

Bonner, R. L., & Rich, A. R. (1987). Toward a predictive model of suicidal behavior: Some preliminary data in college students. *Suicide and Life-Threatening Behavior, 17*(1), 50–63.

Buda, M., & Tsuang, M. (1990). The epidemiology of suicide: Implications for clinical practice. In S. Blumenthal & D. Kupfer (Eds.), *Suicide over the life cycle* (pp. 17–37). Washington, DC: American Psychiatric Press.

Bunney, W., & Fawcett, J. (1965). Possibility of a biochemical test for suicide potential. *Archives of General Psychiatry, 13,* 232–239.

Burns, D. D., & Auerbach, A. (1996). Therapeutic empathy in cognitive behavioral therapy: Does it really make a difference? In P. M. Salkovskis (Ed.), *Frontiers of cognitive therapy* (pp. 135–164). New York: Guilford Press.

Chowdhury, N., Hicks, R., & Kreitman, N. (1973). Evaluation of an after-care service for parasuicide (attempted suicide patients). *Social Psychiatry, 8,* 67–81.

Clark, D. A. (1995). Perceived limitations of standard cognitive therapy: A consideration of efforts to revise Beck's theory and therapy. *Journal of Cognitive Psychotherapy: An International Quarterly, 9,* I153–I172.

Clark, D., & Fawcett, J. (1992). Review of empirical risk factors for evaluation of the suicidal patient. In B. Bongar (Ed.), *Suicide: Guidelines for assessment, management, and treatment* (pp. 16–48). New York: Oxford University Press.

Clark, D., Young, M., Scheftner, W., Fawcett, J., & Fogg, L. (1987). A field-test of Motto's risk estimator for suicide. *American Journal of Psychiatry, 144,* 923–926.

Craighead, L., Craighead, W., Kazdin, A., & Mahoney, M. (1994). *Cognitive and behavioral interventions: An empirical approach to mental health problems.* Boston: Allyn & Bacon.

Craighead, W., & Craighead, L. (1998). Manual-based treatments: Suggestions for improving their clinical utility and acceptability. *Clinical Psychology: Science and Practice, 5*(3), 404–407.

DiBianco, J. (1979). The hemodialysis patient. In L. Hankoff & B. Einsidler (Eds.), *Suicide: Theory and clinical aspects.* Littleton, MA: PSG.

Dowd, E. T., & Courchaine, K. E. (1996). Implicit learning, tacit knowledge, and implications for stasis and change in cognitive psychotherapy. *Journal of Cognitive Psychotherapy, 10*(3), 163–180.

Dublin, L. (1963). *Suicide: A sociological and statistical study.* New York: Ronald.

Durkheim, E. (1951). *Suicide: A study in sociology* (J. A. Spaulding & G. Simpson, Trans.). Glencoe, IL: Free Press. (Original work published 1897)

Ellis, T. E., & Ratliff, K. G. (1986). Cognitive characteristics of suicidal and nonsuicidal psychiatric patients. *Cognitive Therapy and Research, 10,* 625–634.

Fawcett, J., Scheftner, W., Fogg, L., Clark, D., Young, M., Hedeker, D., & Gibbons, R. (1990). Time-related predictors of suicide in major affective disorder. *American Journal of Psychiatry, 147,* 1189–1194.

Freeman, A., & Reinecke, M. (1993). *Cognitive therapy of suicidal behavior.* New York: Springer.

Freud, S. (1957). Mourning and melancholia. In J. Strachey (Ed. and Trans.), *The standard edition of the complete psychological works of Sigmund Freud* (Vol. 4, pp. 237–260). London: Hogarth Press. (Original work published 1917)

Garrison, C. (1992). Demographic predictors of suicide. In R. Maris, A. Berman, J. Maltsberger, & R. Yufit (Eds.), *Assessment and prediction of suicide* (pp. 484–498). New York: Guilford Press.

Gaston, L., Thompson, L., Gallagher, D., Cournoyer, L. G., & Gagon, R. (1998). Alliance, technique, and their interactions in predicting outcome of behavioral, cognitive, and brief dynamic therapy. *Psychotherapy Research, 8,* 190–209.

Gibbons, J., Butler, J., Urwin, P., & Gibbons, J. (1978). Evaluation of a social work service for self-poisoning patients. *British Journal of Psychiatry, 133,* 111–118.

Hagga, D. A., Dyck, M. J., & Ernst, D. (1991). Empirical status of cognitive theory of depression. *Psychological Bulletin, 110,* 215–236.

Hatton, C., Valente, S., & Rink, A. (1977). Assessment of suicide risk. In C. Hatton, S. Valente, & A. Rink (Eds.), *Suicide: Assessment and intervention.* New York Appleton-Century-Crofts.

Hawton, K., Bancroft, J., Catalan, J., Kingston, B., Stedeford, A., & Welch, N. (1981). Domiciliary and outpatient treatment of self-poisoning patients by medical and non-medical staff. *Psychological Medicine, 11,* 169–177.

Hawton, K., McKeown, S., Day, A., Martin, P., O'Connor, M., & Yule, J. (1987). Evaluation of outpatient counseling compared with general practitioner care following overdoses. *Psychological Medicine, 17,* 751–761.

Hendin, H. (1964). *Suicide in Scandinavia.* New York: Grune & Stratton.

Hirsch, S., Walsh, C., & Draper, R. (1983). The concept and efficacy of the treatment of parasuicide. *British Journal of Clinical Psychopharmacology, 15,* 189S–194S.

Hollon, S. D., & Beck, A. T. (1979). Cognitive therapy in depression. In P. C. Kendall & S. D. Hollon (Eds.), *Cognitive-behavioral interventions: Theory, research, and procedures* (pp. 153–203). New York: Academic Press.

Hollon, S. D., & Beck, A. T. (1993). Cognitive and cognitive-behavioral therapies. In A. E. Bergin & S. L. Garfield (Eds.), *Handbook of psychotherapy and behavior change: An empirical analysis* (4th ed., pp. 428–466). New York: Wiley.

Jobes, D. A., & Berman, A. L. (1993). Suicide and malpractice liability: Assessing and revising policies, procedures, and practice in outpatient settings. *Professional Psychology: Research and Practice, 24,* 91–99.

Jobes, D. A., Eyman, J. R., & Yufit, R. I. (1990). *Suicide risk assessment survey.* Paper presented at the annual meeting of the American Association of Suicidology, New Orleans.

Jobes, D. A., & Maltsberger, J. T. (1995). The hazards of treating suicidal patients. In M. Sussman (Ed.), *A perilous calling: The hazards of psychotherapy practice* (pp. 200–214). New York: Wiley.

Joiner, T. E., & Rudd, M. D. (2000). Intensity and duration of suicidal crises vary as a function of previous suicide attempts and negative life events. *Journal of Consulting and Clinical Psychology.* In press.

Joiner, T. E., Rudd, M. D., & Rajab, M. H. (1998). Agreement between self and clinician-rated suicidal symptoms in a clinical sample of young adults: Explaining discrepancies. *Journal of Consulting and Clinical Psychology.*

Kendall, P. (1998). Directing misperceptions: Researching the issues facing manual-based treatments. *Clinical Psychology: Science and Practice, 5*(3), 396–399.

Kleespies, P. (1993). Stress of patient suicidal behavior: Implications for interns and training programs in psychology. *Professional Psychology: Research and Practice, 24,* 477–482.

Kraeplin, E. (1915). *Textbook of psychiatry.* (Original work published 1883)

Lambert, M. (1998). Manual-based treatment and clinical practice: Hangman of life or promising development? *Clinical Psychology: Science and Practice, 5*(3), 391–395.

Lambert, M., & Okiishi, J. (1997). The therapist's contribution to psychotherapy outcome. *Clinical Psychology: Science and Practice, 4,* 66–75.

Layden, M. A., Newman, C. F., Freeman, A., & Morse, S. B. (1993). *Cognitive therapy of borderline personality disorder.* Needham Heights: Allyn & Bacon.

Lerner, M., & Clum, G. (1990). Treatment of suicide ideators: A problem-solving approach. *Behavior Therapy, 21,* 403–411.

Liberman, R., & Eckmen, T. (1981). Behavior therapy vs. insight-oriented therapy for repeated suicide attempters. *Archives of General Psychiatry, 38,* 1126–1130.

Linehan, M. (1981). *Suicidal behaviors questionnaire.* Unpublished inventory, University of Washington, Seattle, WA.

Linehan, M. (1993). *Cognitive-behavioral treatment of borderline personality disorder.* New York: Guilford Press.

Linehan, M. (1997). Behavioral treatments of suicidal behaviors. In D. M. Stoff & J. J. Mann (Eds.), *The neurobiology of suicidal behavior* (pp. 302–328). New York: Annals of the New York Academy of Sciences.

Linehan, M., Armstrong, H., Suarez, A., Allmon, D., & Heard, H. (1991). Cognitive-behavioral treatment of chronically parasuicidal borderline patients. *Archives of General Psychiatry, 48,* 1060–1064.

Linehan, M., Camper, P., Chiles, J., Strosahl, K., & Shearin, E. (1987). Interpersonal problem-solving and parasuicide. *Cognitive Therapy and Research, 11,* 1–12.

Litman, R. (1990). Suicides: What do they have in mind? In D. Jacobs & H. Brown (Eds.), *Suicide: Understanding and responding* (pp. 143–156). Madison, CT: International Universities Press.

Litman, R., & Wold, C. (1976). Beyond crisis intervention. In E. Shneidman (Ed.), *Suicidology: Contemporary developments* (pp. 528–546). New York: Grune & Stratton.

London, P. (1986). Major issues in psychotherapy integration. *International Journal of Eclectic Psychotherapy, 5*(3), 211–216.

MacKinnon, D., & Farberow, N. (1975). An assessment of the utility of suicide prediction. *Suicide and Life-Threatening Behavior, 6,* 86–91.

Mahoney, M. J. (1988). Constructive metatheory: II. Implications for psychotherapy. *International Journal of Personal Construct Psychology, 1,* 299–316.

Maltsberger, J. (1986). *Suicide risk: The formulation of clinical judgement.* New York: New York University Press.

Maltsberger, J. T., & Buie, D. H. (1974). Countertransference hate in the treatment of suicidal patients. *Archives of General Psychiatry, 30,* 625–633.

Maltsberger, J. T., & Buie, D. H. (1989). Common errors in the management of suicidal patients. In D. Jacobs & H. N. Brown (Eds.), *Suicide: Understanding responding.* Madison, CT: International Universities Press.

Maris, R. (1991). The developmental perspective of suicide. In A. Leenaars (Ed.), *Lifespan perspectives of suicide: Time-lines in the suicide process* (pp. 25–38). New York: Plenum.

Maris, R. (1992). The relationship of nonfatal suicide attempts to completed suicide. In R. Maris, A. Berman, J. Maltsberger, & R. Yufit (Eds.), *Assessment and prediction of suicide* (pp. 362–380). New York: Guilford Press.

Maris, R., Berman, A., Maltsberger, J., & Yufit, R. (Eds.). *Assessment and prediction of suicide.* New York: Guilford Press.

McLeavey, B. C., Daly, R. J., Ludgate, J. W., & Murray, C. M. (1994). Interpersonal problem solving skills training in the treatment of self-poisoning patients. *Suicide and Life-Threatening Behavior, 24,* 382–394.

Miller, I., Norman, W., Bishop, S., & Dow, M. (1986). The Modified Scale for Suicide Ideation: Reliability and validity. *Journal of Consulting and Clinical Psychology, 54*(5), 724–725.

Moeller, H. (1989). Efficacy of different strategies of aftercare for patients who have attempted suicide. *Journal of the Royal Society of Medicine, 82,* 643–647.

Montgomery, S., & Montgomery, D. (1982). Pharmacological prevention of suicidal behavior. *Journal of Affective Disorders, 4,* 291–298.

Montgomery, D., Roy, & Montgomery, S. (1981). Mianserin in the prophylaxis of suicidal behavior: A double blind placebo controlled trial. In *Depression and suicide* (Proceedings of the 11th Congress of Suicide Prevention, pp. 786–790). New York: Pergamon Press.

Morgan, H., Jones, E., & Owen, J. (1993). Secondary prevention of non-fatal deliberate self-harm: The green card study. *British Journal of Psychiatry, 163,* 111–112.

Motto, J. (1976). Suicide prevention for high-risk persons who refuse treatment. *Suicide and Life-Threatening Behavior, 6*(4), 223–230.

Motto, J. (1979). The psychopathology of suicide: A clinical approach. *American Journal of Psychiatry, 136*(4-B), 516–520.

Motto, J., Heilbron, D., & Juster, R. (1985). Development of a clinical instrument to estimate suicide risk. *American Journal of Psychiatry, 142,* 680–686.

Murphy, G. (1972). Clinical identification of suicide risk. *Archives of General Psychiatry, 27,* 356–359.

Murphy, G. (1983). On suicide prediction and prevention. *Archives of General Psychiatry, 40,* 343–344.

Murphy, G. (1984). The prediction of suicide: Why is it so difficult? *American Journal of Psychotherapy, 38,* 341–349.

Murphy, G., & Wetzel, R. (1990). The lifetime risk of suicide in alcoholism. *Archives of General Psychiatry, 47,* 383–392.

Nathan, P. (1998). Practice guidelines: Not yet ideal. *American Psychologist, 53*(3), 290–299.

National Institute of mental Health (1998). *Suicide facts.* Internet site: www.nimh.gov/research/suifact.htm.

Neuringer, C. (1968). Divergencies between attitudes towards life and death among suicidal, psychosomatic, and normal hospitalized patients. *Journal of Consulting and Clinical Psychology, 32,* 59–63.

Neuringer, C., & Lettieri, D. J. (1971). Cognition, attitude, and affect in suicidal individuals. *Suicide and Life-Threatening Behavior, 1,* 106–124.

Newman, C. (1997). Maintaining professionalism in the face of emotional abuse from clients. *Cognitive and Behavioral Practice, 4*(1), 1–29.

Newman, C. F. (1994). Understanding client resistance: Methods for enhancing motivation to change. *Cognitive and Behavioral Practice, 1*(7), 47–69.

Nezu, A., Nezu, C., & Perri, M. (1989). *Problem-solving therapy for depression: Theory, research, and clinical guidelines.* New York: Wiley.

O'Carroll, P., Berman, A., Maris, R., Moscicki, E., Tanney, B., & Silverman, M. (1996). Beyond the tower of Babel: A nomenclature for suicidology. *Suicide and Life-Threatening Behavior, 26,* 237–252.

Orbach, I. (1997). A taxonomy of factors related to suicidal behavior. *Clinical Psychology: Science and Practice, 4,* 208–224.

Orbach, I., Rosenheim, E., & Harry, E. (1987). Some aspects of cognitive in suicidal children. *Journal of the American Academy of Child and Adolescent Psychiatry, 26,* 181–185.

Patsiokas, A., & Clum, G. (1985). Effects of psychotherapeutic strategies in the treatment of suicide attempters. *Psychotherapy, 22*(2), 281–290.

Patsiokas, A., & Clum, G., & Luscomb, R. (1979). Cognitive characteristics of suicide attempters. *Journal of Consulting and Clinical Psychology, 47,* 478–484.

Patterson, W., Dohn, H., Bird, J., & Patterson, G. (1983). Evaluation of suicidal patients: The SAD PERSON scale. *Psychosomatics, 24,* 343–349.

Paykel, E. S., Myers, J. K., Lindenthal, J. J., & Tanner, J. (1974). Suicidal feelings in the general population: A prevalence study. *British Journal of Psychiatry, 124,* 460–469.

Persons, J. (1995). Are all psychotherapies cognitive? *Journal of Cognitive Psychotherapy, 9*(3), 185–194.

Persons, J., Thase, M., & Crits-Christoph, P. (1996). The role of psychotherapy in the treatment of depression. *Archives of General Psychiatry, 53,* 283–290.

Pokorny, A. (1983). Prediction of suicide in psychiatric patients: Report of a prospective study. *Archives of General Psychiatry, 40,* 249–257.

Pokorny, A. (1992). Prediction of suicide in psychiatric patients: Report of a prospective study. In R. Maris, A. Berman, J. Maltsberger, & R. Yufit (Eds.), *Assessment and prediction of suicide* (pp. 105–129). New York: Guilford Press.

Pope, K., & Tabachnick, B. (1993). Therapists' anger, fear, and sexual feelings: National survey of therapist responses, client characteristics, critical events, formal complaints, and training. *Professional Psychology: Research and Practice, 24,* 142–152.

Prezant, D. W., & Neimeyer, R. A. (1988). Cognitive predictors of depression and suicide ideation. *Suicide and Life-Threatening Behavior, 18*(3), 259–264.

Ranieri, W. F., Steer, R. A., Lavrence, T. I., Rissmiller, D. I., Piper, G. E., & Beck, A. T. (1987). Relationship of depression, hopelessness, and dysfunctional attitudes to suicide ideation in psychiatric patients. *Psychological Reports, 61,* 967–975.

Reber, A. S. (1992). An evolutionary context for the cognitive unconscious. *Journal of Philosophical Psychology, 5,* 33–51.

Rice, R., & Jobes, D. A. (1997, April). *Suicide, malpractice, and HMO's.* Paper presented at the meeting of the American Association of Suicidology, Memphis, TN.

Richman, J. (1986). *Family therapy for suicidal individuals.* New York: Springer.

Roth, A., & Fonagy, P. (1996). *What works for whom?: A critical review of psychotherapy research.* New York: Guilford Press.

Rotheram-Borus, M. I., & Trautman, P. D. (1988). Hopelessness, depression, and suicidal intent among adolescent suicide attempters. *Journal of the American Academy of Child and Adolescent Psychiatry, 27,* 700–704.

Roy, A. (1992). Genetics, biology, and suicide in the family. In R. Maris, A. Berman, J.

Maltsberger, & R. Yufit (Eds.), *Assessment and prediction of suicide* (pp. 574–588). New York: Guilford Press.

Rudd, M. D. (1993). Social support and suicide. *Psychological Reports, 72,* 201–202.

Rudd, M. D. (2000). Integrating science into the practice of clinical suicidology: A review of the psychotherapy literature and a research agenda for the future. In R. W. Maris, S. S. Canetto, J. L. McIntosh, & M. M. Silverman (Eds.), *Review of Suicidology, 2000* (pp. 47–83). New York: Guilford Press.

Rudd, M. D., Dahm, P., & Rajab, M. H. (1993). Diagnostic comorbidity in persons with suicidal ideation and behavior. *American Journal of Psychiatry, 150,* 928–934.

Rudd, M. D., & Joiner, T. E. (1997). Countertransference and the therapeutic relationship: A cognitive perspective. *Journal of Cognitive Psychotherapy, 11,* 231–250.

Rudd, M. D., & Joiner, T. E. (1998a). The assessment, management, and treatment of suicidality: Towards clinically informed and balanced standards of care. *Clinical Psychology: Science and Practice, 5*(2), 135–150.

Rudd, M. D., & Joiner, T. E. (1998b). Assessment of suicidality in clinical practice: A framework for outpatient practice. In L. VandeCreek (Ed.), *Innovations in clinical practice* (Vol. 17, pp. 1–17). Sarasota, FL: Professional Resource Press.

Rudd, M. D., Joiner, T. E., Jobes, D. A., & King, C. (1999). The outpatient treatment of suicidality: An integration of science and a recognition of its limitations. *Journal of Professional Psychology: Research and Practice, 30*(5), 437–446.

Rudd, M. D., Joiner, T. E., & Rajab, M. H. (1995). Help negation after acute suicidal crisis. *Journal of Consulting and Clinical Psychology,* 499–503.

Rudd, M. D., Joiner, T. E., & Rajab, M. H. (1996). Relationships among suicide ideators, attempters, and multiple attempters in a young adult sample. *Journal of Abnormal Psychology, 105,* 541–550.

Rudd, M. D., Rajab, M. H., & Dahm, P. (1994). Problem-solving appraisal in suicide ideators and attempters. *American Journal of Orthopsychiatry, 64,* 136–149.

Rudd, M. D., Rajab, H., Orman, D., Stulman, D., Joiner, T., & Dixon, W. (1996). Effectiveness of an outpatient problem-solving intervention targeting suicidal young adults: Preliminary results. *Journal of Consulting and Clinical Psychology, 64,* 179–190.

Safran, J. D., & Greenberg, L. S. (1986). Hot cognition and psychotherapy process: An information processing/ecological perspective. In P. C. Kendall (Ed.), *Advances in cognitive behavioral research and therapy* (Vol. 5, pp. 143–177). Orlando, FL: Academic Press.

Salkovskis, P., Atha, C., & Storer, D. (1990). Cognitive-behavioural problem solving in the treatment of patients who repeatedly attempt suicide: A controlled trial. *British Journal of Psychiatry, 157,* 871–876.

Schotte, D., & Clum, G. (1982). Suicide ideation in a college population: A test of a model. *Journal of Consulting and Clinical Psychology, 50,* 690–696.

Schotte, D., & Clum, G. (1987). Problem-solving skills in suicidal psychiatric patients. *Journal of Consulting and Clinical Psychology, 55,* 49–55.

Schwab, J. J., Warheit, G. J., & Holzer, C. E. III (1972). Suicide ideation and behavior in the general population. *Disorders of the Nervous System, 33,* 745–748.

Seligman, M. (1996). Science as an ally of practice. *American Psychologist, 51,* 1071–1079.

Shneidman, E. (1981). Psychotherapy with suicidal patients. *Suicide and Life-Threatening Behavior, 11*(4), 341–348.

Shneidman, E. (1984). Aphorisms of suicide and some implications for psychotherapy. *American Journal of Psychotherapy, 38*(3), 319–328.

Shneidman, E. (1985). *Definitions of suicide.* New York: Wiley.

Shneidman, E. (1993). *Suicide as psychache: A clinical approach to self-destructive behavior.* Northvale, NJ: Jason Aronson.

Shneidman, E. S. (1987). A psychological approach to suicide. In G. R. Vandenbos & B. K. Bryant (Ed.), *Cataclysms, crises, and catastrophes: Psychology in action* (pp. 147–183). Washington, DC: American Psychological Association.

Shneidman, E. S. (1996). *The suicidal mind.* New York: Oxford University Press.

Silverman, M., Berman, A., Bongar, B., Litman, R., & Maris, R. (1994). Inpatient standards of care and the suicidal patient. Part II: An integration with clinical risk management. *Suicide and Life-Threatening Behavior, 24,* 152–169.

Simon, R. (1987). *Clinical psychiatry and the law.* Washington, DC: American Psychiatric Press.

Simon, R. (1988). *Concise guide to clinical psychiatry and the law.* Washington, DC: American Psychiatric Press.

Slaikeu, K. (1990). *Crisis intervention* (2nd ed.). Boston: Allyn & Bacon.

Somers-Flanagan, J., & Somers-Flanagan, R. (1995). Intake interviewing with suicidal patients: A systematic approach. *Professional Psychology: Research and Practice, 26,* 41–47.

Stromberg, C., Haggarty, D., Leibenluft, R., McMillian, M., Mishkin, B., Rubin, B., & Trilling, H. (1988). *The psychologist's legal handbook.* Washington, DC: Council for the National Register of Health Service Providers in Psychology.

Tanney, B. (1992). Mental disorders, psychiatric patients, and suicide. In R. Maris, A. Berman, J. Maltsberger, & R. Yufit (Eds.), *Assessment and prediction of suicide* (pp. 277–320). New York: Guilford Press.

Termansen, P., & Bywater, C. (1975). S.A.F.E.R.: A follow-up service for attempted suicide in Vancouver. *Canadian Psychiatric Association Journal, 20,* 29–34.

VandeCreek, L., & Knapp, S. (1989). Tarasoff *and beyond: Legal considerations in the treatment of life-endangering patients.* Sarasota: FL: Professional Resource Exchange.

Waterhouse, J., & Platt, S. (1990). General hospital admission in the management of parasuicide: A randomised controlled trial. *British Journal of Psychiatry, 156,* 236–242.

Weishaar, M. (1996). Cognitive risk factors in suicide. In P. Salkovkis (Ed.), *Frontiers of cognitive therapy* (pp. 226–249). New York: Guilford Press.

Weissman, M., Fox, K., & Klerman, G. (1973). Hostility and depression associated with suicide attempts. *American Journal of Psychiatry, 130,* 450–455.

Welu, T. (1977). A follow-up program for suicide attempters: Evaluation of effectiveness. *Suicide and Life-Threatening Behavior, 7(1),* 17–30.

Yufit, R., & Bongar, B. (1992). Suicide, stress, and coping with life cycle events. In R. Maris, A. Berman, J. Maltsberger, & R. Yufit (Eds.), *Assessment and prediction of suicide* (pp. 553–573). New York: Guilford Press.

Index